INDIVIDUAL IDENTIFICATION
and the
LAW ENFORCEMENT OFFICER

INDIVIDUAL IDENTIFICATION
and the
LAW ENFORCEMENT OFFICER

By

DONALD J. NASH, Ph.D.

Professor of Zoology
Colorado State University
Fort Collins, Colorado

With Contributions by

Michael Charney, Ph.D.

Professor of Anthropology
Colorado State University
Fort Collins, Colorado

With a Foreword by

Charles G. Wilber, Ph.D.

Professor of Zoology
Colorado State University
Fort Collins, Colorado
Deputy Coroner
Larimer County, Colorado

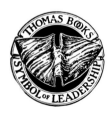

CHARLES C THOMAS · PUBLISHER
Springfield · Illinois · U.S.A

Published and Distributed Throughout the World by

CHARLES C THOMAS • PUBLISHER

Bannerstone House

301-327 East Lawrence Avenue, Springfield, Illinois, U.S.A.

© *1978, by* CHARLES C THOMAS • PUBLISHER

ISBN 0-398-03708-6

Library of Congress Catalog Card Number: 77-24346

*With THOMAS BOOKS careful attention is given to all details of
manufacturing and design. It is the Publisher's desire to present books that
are satisfactory as to their physical qualities and artistic possibilities and
appropriate for their particular use. THOMAS BOOKS will be true to those
laws of quality that assure a good name and good will.*

Library of Congress Cataloging in Publication Data

Nash, Donald J.
　　Individual identification and the law enforcement officer.

　　Bibliography: p.
　　Includes index.
　　1. Identification. 2. Medical jurisprudence.
3. Criminal investigation. I. Charney, Michael,
joint author. II. Title.
HV8073.N29　　　364.12'5　　　77-24346
ISBN 0-398-03708-6

Printed in the United States of America

C-1

Foreword

THE PROBLEM of identification of individuals who are victims of some criminal act, or victims of some disaster caused by nature or man-made operations, or for various other reasons have lost their identification is a complex matter which requires high technical skills and the use of a wide variety of scientific tools.

Professor Nash in this book on individual identification attempts to bring together in a brief form the various practical matters for identifying individuals. To this endeavor Professor Nash brings a wealth of experience and qualifications. He is nationally recognized as one of the leading experimental geneticists in the country. He is known for his study of birth defects resulting from genetic and from environmental factors. He has applied his wealth of knowledge of human heredity to practical problems that one runs into in the criminal justice system.

When all conditions are ideal, it is possible to use the virtually infallible method of fingerprinting to identify individuals. However, in many instances, the fingerprints are unobtainable because of mutilation due to decomposition of the body or as a result of planned removal of hands and feet on the part of some felon. In many instances where clear fingerprints are obtainable, there may be on record no reference set of fingerprints against which one can compare the unknowns. So, despite the fact that fingerprints do indeed provide a positive method of identification, even if everything is just right, there are many instances where other methods must be used.

In this book, Doctor Nash addresses himself to those other methods as well as to the method of fingerprinting. The promise of lipprints is one which must not be overlooked.

The book makes no pretense of being a laboratory manual for the officer who is going to involve himself immediately in the bench-level activities associated with identification. Rather, the book is more broadly focused so that all levels in the criminal justice system can benefit by it. It stresses principles, and it stresses how various methods work and what answers they can give. It is truly a book which can be read profitably by all echelons of the criminal justice system.

This book, if supplemented by an actual laboratory manual, should prove to be an outstanding textbook for individuals who want information on the methodology.

An illustration of the importance of identification comes to mind in the case of unidentified remains recovered from a fire. The first point to ascertain is whether the remains are human. Such determination begins with a complete x-ray examination of the entire remains. Bones and teeth resist the action of fire better than any other part of the body. If an adequate amount of bone is left, it is simple after examination of the x-ray film to arrive at a tentative conclusion concerning the sex and age of the individual. Various kinds of debris, such as buckles, hairpins, zippers, and the like, also will give some kind of indication as to sex of the individual. If any significant amount of bony structure can be recovered from the remains, one can then estimate the height, the weight, and even the build of the person. The determination of race is difficult unless a rather complete skull remains. Teeth, of course, are important in identifying remains down to the individual level. One must never forget that various articles of clothing such as shoes, belts, key rings, and so forth may give a clue to the identity of the individual.

In any case involving an unknown body, an accurate and detailed description is mandatory. Such a description is needed in the process of identification. An adequate description includes the extent of livor mortis, the condition of rigor mortis, signs of decomposition, sex, race, estimated age, height and weight. Various scars and evidence of operations or trauma should be noted. If the remains are that of a male, the presence or absence of circumcision should be noted. Dental charts should be prepared by a competent dentist. Artificial dentures often have a serial number or the actual name of the victim imbedded in the plastic material. Tattoos should be photographed or, if necessary, cut out and preserved. There are certain tattoo experts who can tell the country of origin of the tattoo, the port at which the tattoo was made and, in some instances, the specific artist who did the tattooing. Although fingerprinting of bodies that have been recovered from the water, for example, may require special methods, such techniques are available and should be used as part of the identification process. Again it must be emphasized that clothing and other articles found on or near the remains often contain important information. The size, brand names, vendor's label, laundry marks, and other identifying aspects of articles of clothing should be recorded. Cigarette packages quite often will have a serial number which can tell the approximate time of death or immersion and may even indicate where the package of cigarettes was found.

Quite often the identification process is aided if there is information concerning the approximate time that a body was immersed in water. An examination of the skin will give some information. For example, the fingertips begin to shrivel up or show the "washer woman's characteristics" somewhere between two and four hours after immersion. This shrivelling up of the fingertips is fully developed at the end of twenty-four hours. The skin on the palms of the hands begins to shrivel between twenty-four and forty-eight hours. The shrivelling of the soles of the feet begins at about forty-eight hours. The skin at various parts of the body begins to slip off somewhere between four and eight days, depending upon the water temperature. The skin and the nails can be pulled off in a glovelike fashion somewhere between two and three weeks of immersion. It becomes obvious, then, that identification of an unknown body is a technical process, but it is one which can be done with a high probability of success, assuming that investigators are competent and that they use a battery of the latest methods available for the identification of unknown human remains.

The tragedy in the summer of 1976 associated with the flood through the Big Thompson Canyon in Colorado shows the effectiveness of high-quality identification procedures. In that disaster, over 100 individuals are known to have lost their lives. All bodies that were recovered have been identified and have been disposed of according to law and wishes of next of kin.

The problem was complicated by the wide range of ages involved and the large area over which the bodies were strewn as a result of the flood action. However, it was possible, using modern identification techniques, to arrive at the identification of each set of remains.

Professor Nash brings to the reader's attention in a straightforward, useful way the various devices and procedures that aid in the identification of humans. In view of the fact that aircraft accidents, fires, explosions, floods, and other disasters still plague man, it is important for law enforcement personnel and indeed for all segments of the law enforcement community to be aware of the techniques and possibilities of identification of single remains as well as numerous remains which may result from mass disasters.

The book which Professor Nash has created should prove useful to a wide audience. It is hoped that it will serve as an effective text for a short course in identification to be given to law enforcement personnel and other members of the legal system in the United Stares so that all will have an appreciation of the fact that no set of human remains need go unidentified except under the most unusual circumstances.

CHARLES G. WILBER, Ph.D.

Contents

INDIVIDUAL IDENTIFICATION
and the
LAW ENFORCEMENT OFFICER

CHAPTER I

Introduction

THE LITERATURE of forensic science is filled with unusual applications of science to the identification of individuals. The person who is charged with the identification of an unknown body may have to resort to numerous techniques in order to reach a successful identification. A case described by Stevens (1966) illustrates briefly but elegantly the problems involved in the identification of humans.

The case involved victims in the crash of a small civilian plane. The plane, containing a student pilot and a flight instructor, had crashed into the sea. The body of the student was recovered and identified a few days after the crash, but the instructor was not found. Three and one-half months following the crash, a headless and limbless torso was washed ashore several miles from the site where the student's body had been discovered.

The incomplete nature of the body obviously eliminated many of the usual methods of identification. The corpse was x-rayed, as x-rays of the missing instructor were available from the previous year. The postmortem x-rays of the unknown body had many points of similarity with the antemortem films of the pilot. Stevens mentions that

> the similarities included scoliosis of the spine with slight convexity to the right, maximal at dorsal 8 to 9 level, marked spondylosis of the right eighth and ninth costo-transverse joints, unusually large and shaped tubercles on the first ribs and in particular on the left second rib, and distinctly shaped and splayed left sixth, seventh and eighth ribs.

It was felt that the x-ray comparisons alone were sufficient to make a positive identification. However, an additional line of evidence was available which, although it could not by itself provide identity, did provide a strong contributing force.

Samples of several organs from the unknown body were typed for their ABO blood group system. All samples gave strong group B reactions. Prior to the determinations, the pilot's wife had in-

3

dicated her husband had been blood group B. In the British population, type B occurs at a frequency of 8 in 100. The fact that the unknown had the same blood type as the pilot thus could be considered as an additional step in the direction of a positive identification. Blood groups by themselves may be of limited value in identification but, in cases such as this, may provide evidence for confirmation.

One other important point was raised by Stevens in the above case. He noted that the police had acted surprisingly slowly in seeking pathological or medical assistance in the identification of the body. In effect, they had assumed it was beyond identification. Law enforcement personnel should realize that in difficult cases, different types of medical evidence may lead to a successful identification.

One additional study will be described as an introduction to the ever-fascinating work of individual identification. A most interesting case of identification requiring the utilization of several methods was described by Spitz et al. (1970). The study involved the identification of two individuals killed in an explosion of an automobile. Two bodies were recovered at the scene of the explosion. One of the victims was identified readily on the basis of direct visual identification by relatives and friends. Fingerprints later confirmed the identification of the victim. The second body presented many problems because of the extensive mutilation of the body. There did not appear to be any identifying scars, deformities, or tattoos. Additional interest was generated in the case by the possibility that the second victim might have been H. Rap Brown, a militant black leader due to stand trial.

The efforts to identify the victim included an intense search for fingerprint fragments and a reconstruction of the facial features along with subsequent photographs and drawings of the reconstructed contours. Personal papers found at the scene of the accident also were processed. A follow-up of one of the names found on an identification card and military discharge papers led the search to the military dental records of a William H. Payne. However, the military dental charts of W. H. Payne did not compare with the postmortem dental examination of the blast victim. It was concluded that the two persons were not the same because of the discrepancy in the dental patterns. It should at this time be noted, however, that the blood group of the victim was O+ and was similar to that reported for W. H. Payne.

Considerable effort was directed towards the reconstruction of the facial features. An artist sketched the reconstruction, and a facsimile of the face was prepared with the aid of an Identi-kit®. Photographs of the reconstruction were taken from different angles. The photographs revealed that the frontal hairline was grossly irregular. In addition, there were numerous well-defined areas of alopecia (hairlessness). These areas were scattered throughout the black, coarse, cropped hair.

Comparison of photographs of the left ear of the victim with those of H. Rap Brown revealed discrepancies. The hairlines also revealed some obvious differences.

A detailed search of the scene of the explosion did turn up three fragments of skin, including the right thumb and left little finger. Comparison of prints of two of the fragments with prints of the right thumb and left little finger of W. H. Payne revealed that they were identical. As indicated above, the dental records of the unknown victim had not matched those of Payne. However, the identification of the unknown as Payne was confirmed by personal identification by a friend and members of the family. Two of the features mentioned earlier played a major role in the personal identification. These features were the patches of baldness and the shape of the hairline.

The artist's sketch and Identi-kit reproductions also turned out not to be consistent with the features of the deceased. In spite of the discrepancy in the dental records, it was concluded that the identification of the unknown blast victim was, in fact, Payne.

The above two cases illustrate very well the variety of techniques that may have to be utilized in the identification of individuals. The techniques include examination of the skeleton, teeth, blood groups, fingerprints, personal appearance identification, drawings, Identi-kits, and hair. The remainder of this book will be devoted to an examination of these methods as well as some others. The case described by Stevens also emphasizes the point that good techniques in the hands of the inexperienced or the careless experienced worker can lead to erroneous results and conclusions. Where so much may be at stake in the identification of individuals, there is no substitute for carefully thought-out, meticulous procedures.

CHAPTER 2

The Biological Basis of Individual Uniqueness

Most persons are fully aware that no two individuals ever seem to be exactly alike. Human beings, not only among different populations around the world but also within even a relatively homogeneous population, differ from each other in a variety of features. The uniqueness of individuals includes physical, biochemical, psychological, and behavioral features. Even in the case of identical twins, who may appear virtually identical at first glance, detailed observation and familiarization soon establish differences. Philosophers for a long time have written extensively about the importance and significance of the individual. The great advances in the biological sciences during the past century have served to underscore the biological nature of individuals. Numerous books and treatises attest to this philosophical and biological vein, including *The Uniqueness of Individuals* by the British biologist and Nobel Prize winner Sir Peter B. Medawar. Individual identification, on whatever basis is used, relies on the above observations and rests on the most important assumption that every human being is, in fact, unique.

Since the uniqueness of each person is the key to successful identification, it would be well to examine briefly the means by which such uniqueness is achieved. It would be impossible to identify and isolate all the factors and influences that shape a living organism. An answer to the question "What is the basis of individual uniqueness?" can be expressed easily in general terms, but complete understanding remains one of the most difficult and most fascinating areas of contemporary biological research. Unfortunately, the law enforcement officer often is faced with seeking out and identifying individuals on the basis of partial pieces or clues to identity.

Development of the Individual

The appearance of an individual is a result of a combination of genetic and environmental forces acting upon him from the

7

time of conception. Each individual commences his development from a fertilized egg or zygote in which is provided the genetic framework or blueprint which will set the limits as to the range of potential characteristics which the individual will develop. The sperm from the father and the egg or ovum from the mother, which together form the zygote or fertilized egg, contain equal amounts of genetic information so that an individual's genetic heritage is provided in equal amounts from both the mother and the father. People thus possess features of both parents, and resemblances may be seen on both sides of the family. Often, as a result of the specific genetic factors that are involved, a person may show a much more pronounced resemblance to one parent than to the other.

The appearance of an individual, whether it be his entire nature or some specific aspect of his physical, physiological, or behavioral makeup, is referred to as his phenotype. Many human traits and individual differences are known to be governed by genetic factors or can be said to have an inborn basis. The genetic constitution of an individual is referred to as his genotype. Some genetic traits, such as eye color, blood types, albinism, fingerprints, the ability to roll one's tongue, and many others, are modified little if at all by the environmental conditions in which the person is raised. Other traits, which also may have a genetic basis, may be markedly influenced and modified by a variety of environmental factors. For example, concerning weight, two persons may both have a genetic predisposition to be heavy. If one has been on an extremely restricted diet and the other on a copious diet, the resulting phenotypes (in this case, body weights) are likely to be quite different. There are thus numerous ways in which hereditary and environmental factors may interact with each other. Geneticists have tried to emphasize the importance of this interaction—as Medawar (1957) has so aptly put it, "Heredity proposes and development disposes." The end result is that human traits may show an almost endless variety of form and thus lead to the vast variation of individuals.

The Genetic Material—Genes and Chromosomes

The genetic material consists of molecules of nucleic acid which are contained within the nucleus of every cell of the body.

The genetic material can be considered to be organized into units called genes. These genes are themselves organized into larger groupings called chromosomes. The chromosomes, as well as the genes contained in them, occur in pairs in the zygote from which a new individual will develop. The number of chromosomes in man in the zygote, as well as in most cells in the adult, is forty-six and is referred to as the diploid or 2N number. The ovum and sperm each contain the haploid or 1N number, or twenty-three chromosomes. Each person has received one set of chromosomes from the mother via the ovum and one set from the father via the sperm. Thus, the chromosomal number is kept constant from generation to generation, being maintained as 2N in all cells except the sex cells, in which the number is reduced to 1N and then the 2N number is restored at fertilization through the union of ovum and sperm.

Utilizing relatively easy technical procedures, it is possible to obtain slides of human chromosomes. For detailed examination of the chromosomes, photographs are taken, and after enlargement, the chromosomes are cut out and positioned in pairs in descending order of length. This systematic arrangement of the chromosomes is termed a karyotype. In man, the forty-six chromosomes (or twenty-three pairs) fall into seven general classes based on the size of the chromosomes and on the position of the centromere, which appears as a constricted region along the axis of the chromosomes.

Certain individual differences can be traced directly to differences in the number and/or kinds of chromosomes. For example, of the twenty-three pairs of chromosomes of each cell, one pair contains genes which determine the primary sexual features of the individual. In the female, the members of this pair of chromosomes (the so-called X or sex chromosomes) are of equal size (Fig. 1). The other twenty-two pairs of chromosomes are called autosomes. In the male, there also are twenty-two pairs of autosomes and one pair of sex chromosomes. However, in the male, unlike the female, the members of the pair of sex chromosomes are unequal in size. One member of the pair is similar in size to the X chromosome of the female, and the other, the Y chromosome, is much smaller (Fig. 2). It is possible to determine the sex of a normal individual from the karyotype alone, females having twenty-two pairs of autosomes and one pair of X chromosomes and males having twenty-two pairs of autosomes and an XY pair. As a result of "mistakes" occurring during the formation of the sex cells or after the fertilized egg has commenced division, resulting cells may end up with abnormal chromosomal numbers. A variety of different phenotypic abnormalities and malformations are known in humans which are due to

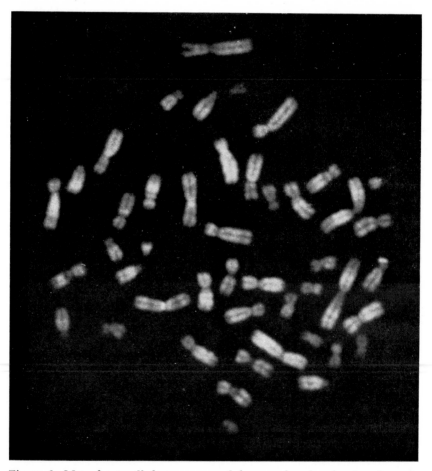

Figure 1. Metaphase cell from a normal human female, showing forty-six chromosomes including one pair of X chromosomes. Photograph by Daniel Chavez.

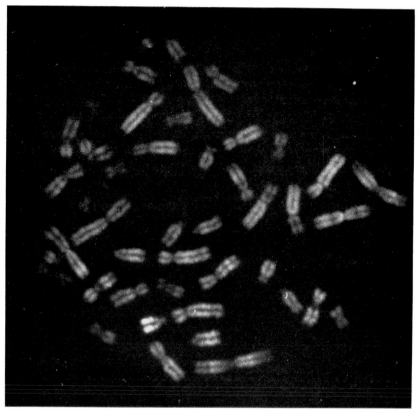

Figure 2. Metaphase cell from a normal human male, also showing forty-six chromosomes but differing from the female cell in that there is only one X chromosome and there also is one Y chromosome. Photograph by Daniel Chavez.

chromosomal abnormalities, including such well-known defects as Down's syndrome, Turner's syndrome, Klinefelter's syndrome, and the XYY condition.

Genetic Variation

During the formation of the sperm or egg cells the twenty-three pairs of chromosomes separate independently of each other. In other words, the set of chromosomes originally furnished by the mother and the set furnished by the father are not inherited together, but the pairs of chromosomes can separate in any combination. In the human with twenty-three pairs of chromosomes, there are over 8 million possible combinations of chromosomes in the formation of the egg or sperm. Looking at this variation in another way, it would mean that the chance of two brothers having received the same combination of chromosomes from their parents is 1 out of 64 million.

However, the genetic variation that is possible as a result of the independent separation of the twenty-three pairs of chromosomes during the formation of the germ cells is by no means the only source of genetic variation. Considering the genes that are located on some particular pair of chromosomes, they may be similar or quite often they may be of a variant or alternative form for some specific trait. It is estimated that in the human, on the average, individuals are variant or heterozygous for 30 percent of their genes. When one considers that there are over 100,000 genes in man, it may be realized that the likelihood of any person producing genetically identical sperm or egg is for all practical purposes zero.

Are Identical Twins Identical?

The closest thing to an exception to the generality that no two people possess the same genetic information would occur in the case of identical twins. Identical or monozygotic twins come about as a result of a single fertilized ovum having split early in development into two parts. Each part receives a complete set of genetic information which is identical in each part. In this sense, the two cells which are theoretically destined to develop into two identical twins are initially identical. However, in the course of development from the one-cell stage to the time of birth, various genetic and environmental factors may exert their influences so that what may have been programmed to be genetically identical may come to differ in appearance. Mutations or changes in the genetic information may occur and cause even the "identical" twins to not be genetically identical. Subtle maternal influences may also operate during development to cause differences in the appearance of identical twins. It should be kept in mind that for all individuals, identical twins included, the genes are always operating in some specific environment and that the potential expression of a gene may be markedly influenced by the environment.

Single Gene Inheritance in Man

The usual manner of describing or identifying someone is by specifying certain components or traits of his overall phenotype. A number of phenotypic characteristics are known in humans in which the trait is governed by genetic factors. Of these genetically determined traits, certain of them are governed by so-called simple Mendelian inheritance. That is to say, the pattern of inheritance of the trait can be followed readily in different family histories. A few specific examples of Mendelian inheritance in man may be useful to illustrate the role of heredity in human individuality.

Certain humans have the ability to roll the tongue in a U shape (Fig. 3), whereas others cannot do so. For this particular phenotype then, there are two alternative forms or characteristics—the ability to roll the tongue or the inability to roll the tongue—and people fall into one of these two categories. In the United States, for example, about 70 percent of the people have the ability, whereas 30 percent lack it. The alternative forms of this particular trait are determined by a single pair of genes. The two genes are located at the same spot or region of one of the

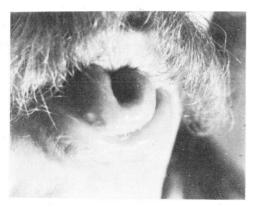

Figure 3. A person demonstrating the ability to roll his tongue into a U shape. *Note:* Recent evidence indicates that this trait may not be inherited in a simple manner.

twenty-three pairs of chromosomes which the human possesses. Each of these locations on the twenty-three pairs of chromosomes is known as a gene locus, and there are thousands of gene loci.

Upon studying the tongue trait in a number of families, a definite pattern of inheritance may be deduced. It turns out that a person who cannot roll his tongue in the above manner has two identical or similar genes at the locus in question. We say that the individual is homozygous for the gene since he bears two copies of the same gene—tt, for example. On the other hand, persons who can roll their tongues turn out to be of two types genetically. They either have two genes which are alike, TT, and phenotypically have the ability to roll, or else they have one gene for the ability and one gene for the inability. In the second case, they are said to be heterozygous for the gene. Since in this specific example the heterozygous genotype Tt has the same phenotype as the homozygous TT, we say that the gene which governs the ability to roll is dominant to the gene responsible for the inability to roll. The latter gene is referred to as a recessive gene.

Referring back to our discussion of chromosomes, an individual receives one each of the two genes from the set of chromosomes that came in from the maternal egg and paternal sperm. Depending on the genotype of an individual (TT, Tt, or tt) and the genotype of his mate, different types of children may result from the different combinations of mating. The two types of homozygous persons can produce only one type of sex cell each. If a person is TT, the sex cells, be they sperm or egg, will contain a chromosome with the T gene. If the person is tt, only the t gene will be present. A heterozygous individual, Tt, will produce two types of sex cells. They will contain either a chromosome containing the T gene or one containing the t gene, and the two types of cells are expected to be produced in equal numbers. As an example, a theoretical pedigree of a human family is shown in Figure 4. Given the pedigree showing phenotypes and based on our knowledge of the genetics of this trait, we can say certain things about the genotypes of the individuals. Since we know that the nonroller phenotype comes about as a result of a

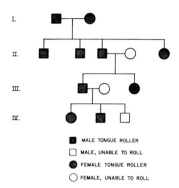

Figure 4. Pedigree of a family in which the tongue-rolling trait is found.

person being homozygous for the t gene, we can assume that all nonrollers have the genotype tt. In the case of the roller phenotype, without any additional knowledge, all we know is that the person must have at least one dominant T gene, since either TT or Tt will give the same phenotype. Looking at the rollers in generations I and II, that is all we can say for certain. Concerning generation III, we could deduce that the male roller must be heterozygous Tt. This would be evident on two counts. First, one of his parents is a nonroller and must have contributed a t gene to his makeup. The second line of evidence comes from the observation that when mated to a nonroller woman, one of their children was a nonroller. The only regular way in which two rollers would have a nonroller child would be if they were, in fact, heterozygous Tt. The roller children in generation IV could be either homozygous TT or heterozygous Tt, but there is no way of telling without additional information.

The above example is a simple demonstration which shows how a knowledge of heredity may help to explain why children resemble their parents for certain traits and why they may be different from one or both parents.

Biology and Genetics of the ABO Blood Groups

As an example of the mechanism of inheritance of a somewhat more complex trait in humans, the ABO blood groups might be discussed. The ABO blood groups have found the widest medicolegal applications of all of the human genetic variants and have been utilized extensively in individual identification in a variety of circumstances.

Three of the four major ABO blood groups were first discovered by Karl Landsteiner in 1900. Doctor Landsteiner often is referred to as the founder or father of serology, the science of the study of blood. In most elementary biology and genetics textbooks, the ABO blood group system is said to consist of three alleles of a single gene, the three alleles being i^A (the "A" gene), i^B (the "B" gene), and i (the "O" gene). Each person receives only one allele from each parent, so that six different combinations of the three alleles are possible in the population. These six combinations are i^Ai^A, i^Ai, i^Bi^B, i^Bi, i^Ai^B, ii. Since these six combinations represent the combinations of genes that individuals may have, they are referred to as genotypes, and specifically in this case, ABO blood group genotypes. The actual "appearance" or phenotype of a person for the ABO blood group trait will depend on which two alleles he has and the relationship of the genes to each other. It turns out that the combination i^Ai has the same phenotype as the combination i^Ai^A. In cases where one gene "masks" the effect of another gene, it is said to be a dominant gene. Thus, i^A is dominant to i, and i is recessive to i^A. Similarly, i^B is dominant to i. When combined in the same individual, i^A and i^B are neither dominant or recessive to each other but produce a distinct phenotype and are said to be codominant. Table I summarizes the possible genotypes and phenotypes utilizing this simplified three-allele model for the ABO blood groups.

Six different genotypes are possible, but only four phenotypes can be recognized, since the genotypes i^Ai^A and i^Ai and the geno-

TABLE I

ABO PHENOTYPES AND GENOTYPES UTILIZING
THREE ALLELES, iA, iB, i

Phenotype (Blood Group)	Genotype	Antigens on Red Cells	Antibodies in Serum
A	iAiA or iAi	A	anti-B
B	iBiB or iBi	B	anti-A
AB	iAiB	A, B	none
O	ii	none	anti-A, anti B

TABLE II

TYPES OF CHILDREN EXPECTED FROM DIFFERENT MATINGS
OF ABO BLOOD GROUP PHENOTYPES AND GENOTYPES

Blood Group Phenotypes	Possible Genotypes	Types of Children Expected Genotypes (Phenotypes in Parentheses)
O × O	$ii \times ii$	ii (O)
O × A	$ii \times i^A i^A$	$i^A i$ (A)
	$ii \times i^A i$	$i^A i$ (A) , ii (O)
O × B	$ii \times i^B i^B$	$i^B i$ (B)
	$ii \times i^B i$	$i^B i$ (B) , ii (O)
O × AB	$ii \times i^A i^B$	$i^A i$ (A) , $i^B i$ (B)
A × A	$i^A i^A \times i^A i^A$	$i^A i^A$ (A)
	$i^A i^A \times i^A i$	$i^A i^A$ (A) , $i^A i$ (A)
	$i^A i \times i^A i$	$i^A i^A$ (A) , $i^A i$ (A) , ii (O)
A × AB	$i^A i^A \times i^A i^B$	$i^A i^A$ (A) , $i^A i^B$ (AB)
	$i^A i \times i^A i^B$	$i^A i^A$ (A) , $i^A i$ (A) , $i^B i$ (B) , $i^A i^B$ (AB)
A × B	$i^A i^A \times i^B i^B$	$i^A i^B$ (AB)
	$i^A i^A \times i^B i$	$i^A i^B$ (AB) , $i^A i$ (A)
	$i^A i \times i^B i^B$	$i^A i^B$ (AB) , $i^B i$ (B)
	$i^A i \times i^B i$	$i^A i^B$ (AB) , $i^A i$ (A) , $i^B i$ (B) , ii (O)
B × B	$i^B i^B \times i^B i^B$	$i^B i^B$ (B)
	$i^B i^B \times i^B i$	$i^B i^B$ (B) , $i^B i$ (B)
	$i^B i \times i^B i$	$i^B i^B$ (B) , $i^B i$ (B) , ii (O)
B × AB	$i^B i^B \times i^A i^B$	$i^A i^B$ (AB) , $i^B i^B$ (B)
	$i^B i \times i^A i^B$	$i^B i^B$ (B), $i^B i$ (B) ,$i^A i$ (A), $i^A i^B$ (AB)
AB × AB	$i^A i^B \times i^A i^B$	$i^A i^A$ (A) , $i^A i^B$ (AB) , $i^B i^B$ (B)

types $i^B i^B$ and $i^B i$ cannot be distinguished by the blood grouping or serological tests. It should be noted at this point, however, that it may be possible to infer what a person's genotype is on the basis of the phenotypes and genotypes of his parents, children, or other relatives. Deductions based on the latter types of knowledge are the basis for the wide use of the ABO blood groups in cases of disputed paternity and in cases of the mistaken identity of children. Under the simplified ABO model presented above, there are ten possible kinds of mating involving the four blood group phenotypes (ignoring the sex of the parent) and twenty-one possible types of mating when the six different genotypes are paired in all possible combinations. Given a certain type of mating of specific genotypes, certain genotypes and phenotypes of children are expected to occur (Table II).

Several important points should be emphasized from this table. For most of the possible kinds of matings of phenotypes or blood groups it is not possible to determine the specific genotypes that are involved for each parent, since some of the genotypes yield the same phenotype. The kinds of children expected for each of the genotypic matings is what would be expected on the average in an infinitely large family. Since human families are, in a genetic sense, of quite limited size and also just due to chance, the kinds of children and the ratios of children expected under a certain mating are not usually found in a single family.

It was stated earlier that the above presentation of the ABO system was simplified. Subgroups of blood group A, for example, have been described, as have several other rare variants. Within the A group the alleles A_1 and A_2 have been reported, with A_1 being dominant to A_2. With just the substitution of these two alleles, the number of phenotypes is increased to six and the number of distinct genotypes to ten. Provided the serological techniques are good, the additional subgroups allow a finer resolution of phenotypes and can increase the powers of individual identification.

Blood Groups and "Disputed Paternity"

In so-called "disputed paternity" cases, the blood group phenotypes of the mother and child are known and some male is suspected or accused of being the father. ABO blood grouping tests of the man in this situation could show either that the man could not possibly be the father or that it might be possible for him to be the father. It is most important to realize that the existence of the second possibility is not anywhere near the same thing as saying that the man *is* the father.

Significance of Genetic Traits in Individual Identification

The various kinds of genetically determined traits may have different degrees of usefulness for the purpose of establishing identity. As indicated earlier, certain characteristics are determined almost exclusively by genetic factors, and the expression of these traits rarely, if ever, is to any extent appreciably modifiable by environmental forces or agents. For example, the utilization of fingerprints as a means of identification is based on the two assumptions: that the set of fingerprints from one individual is distinct from the set of fingerprints of every other individual and that an individual's fingerprints are a permanent characteristic and cannot be altered readily. Other characteristics such as an individual's ABO blood group trait typically are a permanent trait of that individual, but this trait may be shared with millions of other individuals and it may not be possible to associate one particular blood group with a specific individual without resorting to the use of other traits or other kinds of evidence.

Other characteristics of an individual may be altered and modified readily, so that their value alone for individual identification may be virtually worthless. Such traits as weight or hair color, while useful as part of a general description in connection with other physical characteristics, even if they remain a constant trait over a long period of time are nevertheless too common in the general population to stamp the uniqueness of a person. It should be noted, however, that by utilizing a combination of such traits it is possible to narrow the field of people who could fit such a description.

Ideally, from the point of view of law enforcement, any system of individual identification should utilize characteristics that maximize the unique nature of every person, that are easy to measure, that are a permanent trait of the individual, that cannot be modified, at least by simple means, by conscious or subconscious environmental manipulations, and that can be obtained from a variety of kinds of evidence.

CHAPTER 3

Fingerprints and Other Dermal Ridges

THE IMPORTANCE of fingerprints as a means of individual identification is well known by most persons as a result of its numerous applications in story plots for television, movies, plays, and books. In addition, many people have had a direct exposure to fingerprinting in the military service or in applications for driver's licenses. Fingerprinting was one of the earliest methods utilized in scientific crime detection, and it continues to represent one of the most dependable tools available to the forensic scientist.

It is of interest to note the early use of fingerprints as the basis for the plot in "Pudd'nhead Wilson" by Mark Twain. It is remarkable that Twain's story, published in 1895, appeared so soon after the publication, in 1892, of the first scientific treatise by Sir Francis Galton. The following passage is taken from "Pudd'nhead Wilson" and may serve as an interesting and delightful introduction to the "facts" of fingerprints.

> Every human being carries with him from his cradle to his grave certain physical marks which do not change their character, and by which he can always be identified—and that without shade of doubt or question. These marks are his signature, his physiological autograph, so to speak, and this autograph cannot be counterfeited, nor can he disguise it or hide it away, nor can it become illegible by the wear and mutations of time. This signature is not his face—age can change that beyond recognition; it is not his hair, for that can fall out; it is not his height, for duplicates of that exist; it is not his form, for duplicates of that exist also, whereas this signature is each man's very own—there is no duplicate of it among the swarming populations of the globe!
>
> This autograph consists of the delicate lines or corrugations with which nature marks the insides of the hands and the soles of the feet. If you will look at the balls of your fingers,—you that have very sharp eyesight—you will observe that these dainty curving lines lie close together, like those that indicate the borders of oceans in maps and that they form various clearly defined patterns, such as arches, circles, long curves, whorls, etc., and that these patterns differ on the different

Finger Prints, Cummins aptly summarized the contributions of Galton to the science of fingerprinting.

> He brought together and strengthened the evidences essential to the validation of fingerprints as means of personal identification, though none of the concepts was original with him; permanence of the finger-print characteristics; uniqueness of an assemblage of ridge details; variability and classifiability of finger patterns. Furthermore, he reported on fundamental investigations: biological variations as manifested in fingerprints; inheritance of fingerprint traits; variation among racial and constitutional groups. . . . The book is a classic, an outstanding landmark in the progress of fingerprint science.

Different systems of classification of fingerprints have been developed. Edward Richard Henry published his system of classification in book form in 1900, and it is the *Henry System* which forms the basis of our modern system. This system, with a few modifications employed by the FBI, is the system that is utilized today in the classification of fingerprints in the United States.

Biology of Fingerprints

Fingerprints are a result of the pattern of raised strips of skin or ridges which form on the inside of the end joint of the fingers. The ridges begin to form during the third and fourth month of pregnancy and are not necessarily continuous but most of the time are a series of units or islands. The ridges do not change, so that the pattern they form stays the same. Thus, the number of ridges and the patterns which they form are relatively constant and are not obliterated by growth or shrinkage.

Although the initial development and differentiation of the ridges commence about the third month of prenatal life, differentiation is not fully completed until around the seventh month. During this period of differentiation, abnormalities of development may occur and lead to abnormal patterns of the dermal ridges. Abnormal dermatoglyphic patterns are associated with some of the chromosomal disorders of man. In Down's syndrome, for example, a chromosomal disorder in which individuals have forty-seven chromosomes instead of the usual number of forty-six, there are characteristic dermal patterns that aid in

distinguishing patients from unaffected persons. Although there is no one dermal feature that is unique to patients with Down's syndrome, the patients show trends and frequencies of features that distinguish them from normal persons. Walker (1958) demonstrated that, utilizing just dermal patterns alone, about 70 percent of patients with Down's syndrome could be diagnosed. A single transverse crease in the palm, the so-called simian crease, occurs in about half of the patients with Down's syndrome but only occurs in about 1 percent of normal persons. Patients with Down's syndrome also commonly have ulnar loops on all ten fingers and a distal axial triradius on the palm. Since the discovery that Down's syndrome is due to a chromosomal abnormality, interest has developed into studying dermal ridge patterns as an aid in diagnosing many types of chromosomal disorders. The simian crease and distal axial triradius mentioned for Down's syndrome also are frequent in many other syndromes due to chromosomal abnormalities.

Patterns of Dermal Ridges

Even to someone inexperienced in the study of fingerprints, careful examination of fingerprints soon reveals that the dermal ridge patterns do show a tremendous variability. In fact, the novice observer may soon think that there is no simple way to categorize the variation into any manageable system of classification. However, the great majority of fingerprints can be grouped into three major groups or patterns referred to as arches, loops, and whorls. Loops may be further classified as radial or ulnar loops, depending upon whether they open or slant to the radial or ulnar side of the finger.

The classification into arches, loops, and whorls is based on the number of triradii that are present. The triradius usually is located near the lower edge of the fingerprint and consists of points from which the ridges radiate out at angles of 120 degrees in three different directions. By definition, arches have no triradii, loops have one, and whorls have two.

Arches consist of two basic types: plain arches and tented arches. In a plain arch, the ridges pass from one side of the fin-

ger to the other with a slight curve in the center portion of the pattern. The second type of arch, the tented arch, has a central triradius, but the number of ridges between the triradius and the center is zero, as is characteristic of all arches. There are two types of loops. Ulnar loops open or slant to the ulnar side of the finger, and radial loops slant to the radial side of the finger. Whorls may be subdivided into four basic groups: plain, central pocket, double, and accidental. In a plain whorl pattern, there are two deltas and at least one ridge which makes a complete circuit. The central pocket whorl also has two deltas and at least one ridge which makes a complete circular turn. However, an imaginary line drawn between the two deltas does not touch or cross any of the circular ridges within the central pattern area. In the double loop whorl, there are two separate loops and two deltas. The accidental whorl combines two different types of patterns, except for the plain arch, and has two or more deltas. Also, if a pattern did not correspond to one of the accepted categories, it would be classified as "accidental."

Loops and whorls may be classified further by ridge tracing or by obtaining the ridge count. The ridge count is the number of ridges which cut or touch an imaginary line drawn from the triradius to the core of the pattern. There must be a "clear" space between the triradius and the first ridge that is counted; in other words, the triradius is not included in the count. The final ridge also is not included in the count when it forms the core of the pattern. As indicated earlier, an arch by definition has no triradius and therefore would have a ridge count of zero. A loop with one triradius has a ridge count of one. However, with whorls, there are two ridge counts, one from each of its triradii to the corresponding core of the pattern. Usually, in most studies, only the higher count is used.

The total ridge count thus provides an objective, quantitative evaluation of the size of the fingerprint pattern. The ridge count is independent of age. In a general way, the ridge count may also reveal something of the nature of the type of pattern. In general, high ridge counts are associated with either whorls or large loops whereas low ridge counts are associated with small loops.

Persistence of Ridge Patterns

As indicated earlier, an important characteristic of fingerprints for utilization in personal identification is that they do not change in appearance with time. The most comprehensive study of the persistence of ridge patterns is that provided by Galton (1892). His samples included prints that covered the intervals from childhood to boyhood, from boyhood to early manhood, from manhood to about the age of sixty, and from age sixty-seven to age eighty. The intervals cover most of the entire life span of man, and Galton's results demonstrate elegantly and conclusively that fingerprint patterns indeed are permanent.

Galton studied the minute details of different fingers from six different individuals that had prints taken at two different times, covering a range of from nine to thirty-one years between prints. He found a total of 388 points of agreement out of 389 points that were studied and mentions having looked for more than 700 points of comparison with only one exception. The exception was of a ridge that had been split in a child but that had closed up a few years later.

Other isolated cases demonstrating the permanence of fingerprints also have been reported occasionally. Cooke (1962) reported an interesting case of a man in St. Louis, Missouri, who was fingerprinted at the age of 102 and who had matching fingerprints in the file that had been taken in 1905, fifty-seven years earlier!

As further evidence of the permanence of the ridge patterns, Galton mentioned that "the marks on the fingers of many Egyptian mummies, and on the paws of stuffed monkeys, still remain legible, until the time when decomposition actually destroys the last vestiges of tissue." Galton also was quick to point out that it is in the general character of the pattern and in the minutiae that persistence prevails. Measurements of the length and width or other dimensions of the ridges do not remain constant but may change as the fingers grow and change with age, use, and disease.

Superficial injuries to the skin by cuts and burns usually only cause temporary damage to the pattern, and the details of the ridge pattern will be normal after healing. If the injuries are severe enough to leave a permanent scar, they may result in a permanent obliteration or distortion of the ridges. In such cases, identification of the individual would not be possible with the complete destruction of the identifying characteristics. Cummins (1935) has discussed the extent of the efforts that some criminals have gone to in order to destroy their fingerprints. By cutting their fingers or even using acid to burn off the skin, they attempt to obliterate the pattern. However, as long as the area involved is not too extensive or too deeply involved, usually enough regenerative tissue remains to develop enough new tissue to make the pattern discernable.

Variation of Pattern Within a Single Individual

Classification of fingerprints into the three general pattern types of whorls, loops, and arches reveals that the frequencies of the different patterns differ on different fingers and between the left and right hands (Tables III and IV). It may be seen that ulnar loops are the most common pattern on all five fingers, accounting for 64 percent of the total patterns. Arches are the least common pattern, accounting for slightly less than 5 percent of the total. Radial loops show the most variability among the fingers ranging from 0.1 percent on digit V to nearly 25 percent on digit II. As will be seen later, these overall pattern frequencies may be influenced by other factors, including sex and race.

It is of interest to examine the types of patterns that are found among the ten fingers of the same individual. Although

TABLE III

FREQUENCIES OF TYPES OF DIFFERENT FINGERS*

| Digit | Whorls | Loops | | Arches |
		Ulnar	*Radial*	
I	35.41	60.89	0.21	3.49
II	29.47	35.20	24.70	10.62
III	16.37	74.07	2.52	7.03
IV	34.44	62.27	0.98	2.30
V	11.41	87.62	0.11	0.85
Total	25.43	64.02	5.69	4.86

* From Cummins and Midlo (1943).

TABLE IV

PERCENTAGE FREQUENCIES OF THE MAJOR PATTERN TYPES ON THE
FINGERS OF 500 UNRELATED MALES FROM THE UNITED KINGDOM*

| | *Left Hand* | | | | |
	V	IV	III	II	I
Arches	1.40	2.60	6.60	9.40	3.40
Ulnar loops	84.40	63.80	72.80	38.00	66.60
Radial loops	0.00	0.00	4.20	23.00	0.40
Whorls	14.20	33.60	16.40	29.60	29.60
	Right Hand				
	V	IV	III	II	I
Arches	0.40	2.00	5.80	9.60	1.60
Ulnar loops	84.00	47.00	69.20	30.60	58.60
Radial loops	0.40	0.80	3.40	26.60	0.20
Whorls	15.20	50.20	21.60	33.20	39.60

* From Holt (1968).

the same pattern sometimes may be found on all ten fingers, it
is more common to find different patterns on the fingers of one
person. Actually, there is a tendency for the pattern of one finger
to be like the pattern on the other fingers of the same person.
Thompson and Bandler (1973) studied the set of 10 fingerprints
of 592 subjects and observed that the patterns in the same individual tended to be alike. Interesting differences were observed
in the frequencies of the pattern types of the left and right
hands. The frequencies of whorls, ulnar loops, radial loops, and
arches for the left and right hands were 30.2, 65.0, 0.3, and 4.4
percent, and 26.94, 63.0, 4.65, and 5.41 percent, respectively.
Thompson and Bandler compared the distribution of individuals
with 0, 1, 2 . . . 10 patterns of any one type with the distribution
expected of the probability of occurrence of a particular pattern
on any digit is random. Readers are referred to the original
paper for additional details as to methodology.

Fingerprints Differences Between Sexes and Among Races

Although differences in the frequencies of dermatoglyphic
features may be observed between males and females and among
various populations of people, it is not possible to assign an individual to a specific race or sex utilizing only dermatoglyphic features. Table V presents a representative sample of the frequen-

cies of the pattern types in several different populations separated by sex.

Study of the populations indicates that, in general, within the same racial population, females tend to have more arches than do males. In sixteen populations cited by Cummins and Midlo (1943), females had more arches than males in fourteen, more ulnar loops (6/10), fewer whorls (10/15), and fewer radial loops (9/10).

The mean total ridge count also varies between males and females and among the different populations. In the four examples cited in Table V, Australian males and females had the highest ridge counts (160.4 and 148.0, respectively), and the French sample had the lowest (129.4 and 124.2). It is evident that the difference between the sexes also varies among populations, being greatest in the British sample (about 18) and least in the French sample (about 5). Rao (1972) attributes the larger ridge count of males than females in a given population to the presence of a higher frequency of whorls and lower frequency of ulnar loops in males on the average than in females. Males also tend to have a larger ridge count of whorls than do females.

Workers in the fields of human genetics and physical anthropology have attempted to utilize dermatoglyphics as an aid in un-

TABLE V

PATTERN TYPES AND MEAN TOTAL RIDGE
COUNTS IN DIFFERENT POPULATIONS

Population	Sex	Pattern Types in % A	R	U	W	Mean Total Ridge Count	Author
Australian aborigines	M	0.45	1.13	35.08	64.82	160.40	Rao, 1972
	F	2.00	1.25	33.00	64.75	148.00	
Japanese	M	1.70	3.30	45.60	49.50	150.80	Matsunga et al., 1968
	F	1.90	2.60	53.20	42.40	139.20	
French	M	7.20	5.10	55.20	32.40	129.40	Matsunga et al., 1968
	F	7.40	2.20	58.60	58.60	124.20	
British	M	4.30	5.90	61.50	28.30	145.00	Holt, 1968
	F	5.70	4.80	65.40	23.90	127.20	
Negroes	M	5.5	3.3	62.2	28.8	. . . . .	cited in Cummins
	F	8.5	2.2	61.4	27.9	. . . . .	and Midlo, 1943
Efé pygmies	M	15.9	2.8	61.6	19.6	. . . . .	cited in Cummins
	F	17.0	2.0	60.7	19.6	. . . . .	and Midlo, 1943

derstanding relationships among populations. Zavala et al. (1971) studied the finger- and palmprints of eight Mexican Indian groups. They found that there was more variation in the dermatoglyphic features of the Indians than for some of the more simply inherited traits such as blood groups and hemoglobins. They concluded that dermatoglyphics were not as efficient and useful in describing and characterizing human populations as other genetic traits.

Various methods, i.e. pattern-type indices and the pattern intensity index, have been used to compare the frequencies of finger patterns in different populations. Dankmeijer's (1938) arch/whorl index

$$\frac{\text{Total frequency of arches}}{\text{Total frequency of whorls}} \times 100$$

has been used widely. It is based on the fact that a rise in the frequency of arches is usually accompanied by a fall in the frequency of whorls, and vice versa.

The pattern intensity index (Cummins and Steggerda, 1935, and Newman, 1960) is the average number of triradii occurring on fingers per individual. The complexity of patterns increases in the order arch, loop, whorl, and it is accompanied by an increase in the number of triradii. Consequently, a low value of the index indicates a high frequency of arches and a high value a high frequency of whorls.

Srivastava (1972) utilized dermatoglyphic characteristics to compare the Sayyads of Lucknow, Uttar Pradesh, India, with their correligionists living in Afghanistan, Arabia, and Turkey. Examination of the values of Dankmeijer (100 a/w), Fwruhata (100 W/L), and pattern intensity indices did not indicate any consistent dermatoglyphic affinities. The Sayyads had the lowest Dankmeijer index (6.85) and were closest to the Arabs (7.77) in the index. The Fwruhata index indicated the Sayyads (72.55) were closest to the Turks (65.76). With the pattern intensity index, the Sayyads had the highest mean value (13.81), followed by the Nwristanis (13.33), Arabs (13.30), and Turks (12.78). It may be seen from the values above that the different indices fail to demonstrate consistent dermatoglyphic affinities among the populations.

Inheritance

A genetic basis for dermal ridges was recognized by Galton, who noted in 1892 that "some of those who have written on finger marks affirm that they are transmissible by descent, others assert the direct contrary, but no inquiry hitherto appears to justify a definite conclusion. Hence we are justified in assuming that the patterns are partly dependent on constitutional causes, in which case it would indeed be strange if the general law of heredity failed in this particular case."

Since the time of Galton, considerable progress has been made in our understanding of the inheritance of dermal ridge patterns. Cummins and Midlo (1943) reported that

abundant evidence now is at hand to prove that some characteristics of finger prints and of other dermatoglyphic areas are inherited. In preview of this evidence, it may be pointed out that genetic factors have a large share in determining variations of dermatoglyphics, as instanced especially by gradations of similarity observed among individuals having different degrees of relationship. The closest possible genetic relationship is that of monozygotic twins. In their dermatoglyphics, as in other features, the members of monozygotic twin pairs typically present similarities of higher degree than those found in any other comparisons of individuals. A progressive reduction in degree of similarity is demonstrable in comparisons involving lessening relationships. Thus paired siblings and the members of fraternal twin pairs are rarely as similar as the members of monozygotic twin pairs. Parent and child on the average show less resemblance than siblings, unrelated individuals of the same race show still less, while maximum differences are found in comparing persons of different races.

Interest and progress in determining the genetic nature of dermal ridges have continued, and Doctor Sarah B. Holt, in 1968, devoted an entire book, *The Genetics of Dermal Ridges,* to the topic. Doctor Holt wrote, "We still do not know how the patterns are formed by the dermal ridges on fingers, palms, soles and toes are inherited, but in the past twenty years advances have been made in our knowledge of the genetics of other features of ridged skin."

Space does not permit a detailed report of the genetic studies, and the reader is referred to the excellent text and bibliography by Holt. Until recently, the evidence indicated that pattern size, as measured by total ridge count, was strongly influenced by heredity. It was felt that ridge count was determined by a number of genes, each with a relatively small effect, i.e. a polygenetically controlled trait. However, Spence et al. (1973) presented data which "suggests that a single major autosomal locus with two additive alleles may account for over half the variation of the quantitative phenotype absolute finger ridge count."

Regardless of the nature of the genetic factors which control dermatoglyphics, the important feature of dermatoglyphics for individual identification is that the dermal ridge patterns are genetically controlled, are unique to each individual, and are almost completely unaffected by the environment.

Classification of Fingerprints

Fingerprints are classified and filed in the United States through the use of the Henry System, with a few changes and modifications by the Federal Bureau of Investigation. A classification formula is derived based upon the type of patterns and their subdivisions. The subdivisions of the formula include the following:

1. Primary classification
2. Secondary
3. Subsecondary
4. Major division
5. Final classification
6. Key

Key	Major	Primary	Secondary	Subsecondary	Final
7	1	6	U	100	12
	0	18	Ur	ooM	

Figures 5, 6, and 7 show examples of a typical fingerprint card with full classification formula. Only a brief summary of the basis of the various classification subdivisions is provided here. Most of the material has been abridged from the FBI publica-

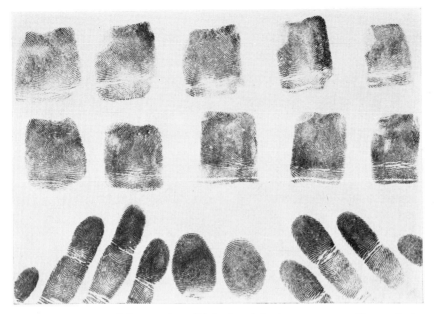

Figure 5. Full set of fingerprints. Right hand is the uppermost line and the right half of the lowest line. Left hand is in the middle and the left half of the lowest line. The order of the fingers in the individual prints from left to right is thumb, index, middle, ring, and little. The classification formula for this set of prints is

$$\frac{6\ 0\ 1\ \text{T}\quad \text{II}\quad 11}{\text{S}\ 17\ \text{U}\ 0\text{II}}$$

Examples of some different patterns are shown by the right thumb (whorl), the right index (tented arch), and the right middle (ulnar loop). Courtesy of Bob Stouffer, Larimer County Sheriff's Department.

tion, "The Science of Fingerprints." Additional details may be found in that book as well as in other standard sources.

Primary Classification

Whorls in any finger are designated by the letter *W*. For the purpose of obtaining the primary classification, values are assigned to each of the ten finger spaces. Wherever a whorl appears, it assumes the value of the space in which it is found. The values are assigned as follows:

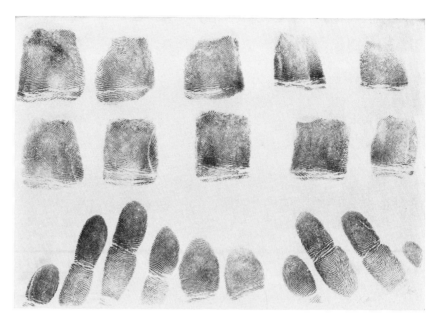

Figure 6. Fingerprints from a male, twenty-three years old and an identical twin to the originator of the prints in Figure 5. Even a casual examination will reveal the extensive differences among the two individuals, who are, of course, genetically most similar. Fingerprints of each person are unique!

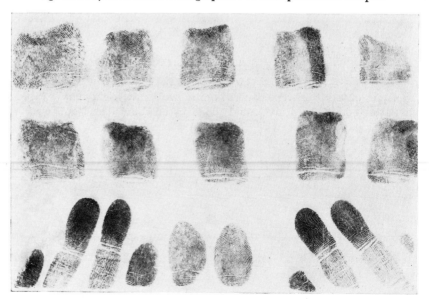

Figure 7. Fingerprints from another person unrelated to the twins. Again note the diversity of the prints within the same individual and among different individuals.

Fingers No. 1 and No. 2 16
Fingers No. 3 and No. 4 8
Fingers No. 5 and No. 6 4
Fingers No. 7 and No. 8 2
Fingers No. 9 and No. 10 . . . 1

Fingers are numbered in the following manner:

1—Right thumb	6—Left thumb
2—Right index	7—Left index
3—Right middle	8—Left middle
4—Right ring	9—Left ring
5—Right little	10—Left little

On the formula, the odd fingers make up the denominator and the even fingers make up the numerator. The sum of the values of the whorl-type patterns, if any, appearing in fingers 1, 3, 5, 7, 9, plus one, is the denominator of the primary. The sum of the values of the whorls, if any, in fingers 2, 4, 6, 8, 10, plus one, is the numerator of the primary.

Secondary Classification

The secondary classification is shown in the formula by capital letters representing the basic types of patterns appearing in the index fingers of each hand, that of the right hand being the numerator and that of the left hand being the denominator. There are five basic types of patterns which can appear.

1. Arch (A)
2. Tented Arch (T)
3. Radial Loop (R)
4. Ulnar Loop (U)
5. Whorl (W)

Prints with an arch or tented arch in any finger or a radial loop in any except the index fingers constitute the lower case letter group of the secondary classification.

Subsecondary Classification

The secondary groups are further subdivided according to the ridge counts of loops and the ridge tracings of whorls. Right hand fingers make up the numerator, left hand fingers make up the denominator. Ridge counts are translated into small and large, represented by Symbols I and O. The whorl tracings are brought up as I, M, or O denoting inner, meeting, or outer ridge tracings of the whorl types. Only six fingers may be involved in the subsecondary—numbers 2, 3, 4, 7, 8, and 9. A ridge count of 1 to 9, inclusive, in the index finger is brought up into the subsecondary formula as I. A count of 10 or more is brought up as O. In the middle fingers, a count of from 1 to 10, inclusive, is brought up as I, and 11 or more is O. In the ring finger, a count of from 1 to 13 is brought up as I, and 14 or more is O.

Major Division

The major division is derived from the patterns occurring in both thumbs. Where whorls appear in the thumbs, the major division reflects the whorl tracings just as the subsecondary does, either as I, M, or O. For loops appearing in thumbs, a table is needed as follows.

Left Thumb Denominator	*Right Thumb Numerator*
1 to 11, inclusive, S (small)	1 to 11, inclusive, S (small)
	12 to 16, inclusive, M (medium)
	17 or more ridges, L (large)
12 to 16, inclusive, M (medium)	1 to 11, inclusive, S (small)
	12 to 16, inclusive, M (medium)
	17 or more ridges, L (large)
17 or more ridges, L (large)	1 to 17, inclusive, S (small)
	18 to 22, inclusive, M (medium)
	23 or more ridges, L (large)

Final Classification

The final classification is based upon the ridge count of the loop on the right little finger. If a loop does not appear in the right little finger, a loop in the left little finger may be used. A ridge count of a whorl pattern occurring on the right little finger may also be obtained if no loops appear on either of the little fingers.

Key

The key is the ridge count of the first loop appearing in a set of prints, beginning with the right thumb but not utilizing the ridge count of any loops which might appear on little fingers.

Identification

In order to establish an identification based upon fingerprints, it is necessary to compare the print in question with other prints having a similar classification. Fingerprint records are filed in such a way that all those prints having the same classification are

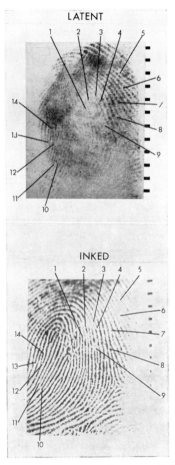

Figure 8. A latent print from a left little finger and the inked print from a suspect later convicted of a burglary. Fourteen points of similarity are demonstrated in the comparison. Readers may pick out additional points. Photographs by Bob Stouffer.

together. Thus, the print being searched is compared only with the groups having a comparable classification rather than with the whole file.

To establish identity, it is necessary to locate several points of identity among the characteristics of the prints. In the United States, twelve corresponding points are generally required as proof of identity, although some American courts have accepted fewer (Fig. 8).

Several key problems are associated with the searching of fingerprint reference files. Although a single print is sufficient to identify its owner, classifying it is a problem and there is no universally accepted method of classifying individual prints. A "10-1" single fingerprint system has been utilized by some law enforcement agencies. This system is a manual approach to fingerprint identification through comparison with latent prints. However, the system is very time consuming and is not very practical for even moderately large collections. Recently, automated equipment has been developed to deal with this problem. Systems such as the Kodak Miracode II® microfilm system and the 3-M Company Microdisc® system have been utilized. These systems can store, search, and retrieve fingerprint cards and other stored information. The machines will automatically eliminate all other data not fitting the descriptors entered by the person making the inquiry.

Automated Fingerprint Identification

In recent years, some progress has been made in developing procedures for identifying and matching fingerprints with the aid of computers. The system does not use the standard features of arches, loops, and whorls which are used in the conventional systems of classification. Instead, fingerprints are classified according to their ridge endings and bifurcations. A photograph of a print can be scanned electronically, analyzed according to its ridge endings, bifurcations, and the position of these features, and the information can then be recorded numerically. The description of a new print can be compared by computer with the "library" of prints that are stored on tape in the computer. According to Wegstein (1970), "it is claimed that the system can identify any filed fingerprints that contain among their total defining information, any position or part that corresponds to the coded information from the crime print. Even a fragment of a print can be analyzed in this way." /

Readers are referred to the work of Wegstein for a more detailed technical description of the procedures involved. The system appears to offer much promise, and it would appear to be only a matter of time before a reliable, totally automated system of fingerprint identification becomes operational. Problems still remain, however, and Wegstein has summarized the sources of difficulty into the following categories:

1. Poor quality prints.

   Prints accepted for classification in the Henry system need to be only clear enough so that a fingerprint expert can identify the pattern type and count the ridges between core and delta. However, it will probably be more effective to change the rules and require higher quality prints for an automated identification system than are required for the Henry system.

2. Only a partial print available.

   It is anticipated that minutiae data from partial prints and particularly latent fingerprints will be usable.

3. A stretched or twisted print.

   No problem due to flexing and twisting in rolled prints.

4. Print displaced in reader in X and Y directions.

   Can be handled by the matches with suitable parameter adjustments.

5. Print rotated in reader.

6. Reader falsely reports minutiae.

7. Reader misses minutiae.

Numbers 6 and 7 tend to increase as the quality of the print goes down.

Dermatoglyphics of Other Areas

It was mentioned earlier that fingerprints are not the only dermal ridges that are utilized in individual identification. The flexion creases of the palms and soles also are of value in identification.

Although its usage is likely to be quite limited, personal identification by means of lipprints (Fig. 9) appears to have a place in forensic science. Suzuki and Tsuchihashi (1970) and Tsuchihashi (1974) have investigated the use of lipprints for personal identification and have done basic studies on individual variations, possible variations with time in the same individual, and some hereditary studies. The paper by Suzuki and Tsuchihashi also furnishes a case report on criminal identification.

Without going into great detail, the classification set up by the Japanese workers is as follows:

Type   I: Clear-cut grooves running vertically across the lip.

Type   I': The grooves are straight but disappear halfway instead of covering the entire breadth of the lip.

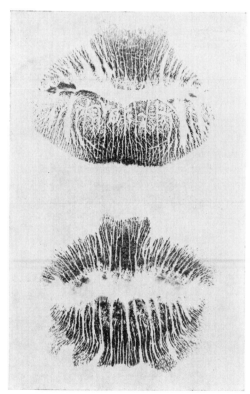

Figure 9. Lipprints from identical female twins, thirty-seven years old.

Type   II: The grooves fork in their course.

Type III: The grooves intersect.

Type IV: The grooves are reticulate.

Type   V: The grooves do not fall into any of the Types I-IV and cannot be differentiated morphologically.

The term *sulci labiorum rubrorum* was coined for the grooves and wrinkles of the lips, and the figure formed by the sulci is called *figura linearum labiorum*. Individual lipprints are recorded in a way similar to a dental formula, by separating the left and right sides of the lip as well as the upper and the lower lips. Examples of two such "formulae" are as follows:

$$\frac{\text{III} \ \text{II} \quad \text{II} \ \text{III}}{\text{II} \ \text{I}' \ \text{I} \quad \text{I} \ \text{I}' \ \text{II}} \ \text{and} \ \frac{\text{II} \ \text{I} \quad \text{I} \ \text{II}}{\text{II} \ \text{I}'\text{I} \quad \text{I} \ \text{I}' \ \text{II}}$$

In this study of 1,364 Japanese subjects, no lipprint showed the same pattern. Also, no individual changes were observed over a three-year period, indicating a relative constancy of pattern. Studies with identical and fraternal twins showed that lipprint patterns of identical twins were much more similar than those of fraternal twins, indicating genetic control of the basic patterns. However, even identical twins did not have exactly identical patterns.

In the case report described by Suzuki and Tsuchihashi (1970), a bomb warning letter mailed to the Tokyo Metropolitan Police Department had two lipprints on the envelope. Lipprints of two suspects were taken, and results demonstrated that the lipprints on the envelope were not made by the two suspects.

CHAPTER 4

Voiceprint Identification

THE EASE WITH WHICH we can identify another individual solely by means of his voice is demonstrated often in our daily lives. In many cases a single word, such as "Hello," spoken on the telephone is enough to reveal the identity of the speaker. Even in cases of individuals whom we have not seen or heard in years, the voice often is distinctive enough for recognition purposes. The above everyday observations have focused attention on the possibility of using an individual's voice as a means of identification.

With the rising number of such crimes as bomb threats, kidnap ransom calls, and obscene phone calls in recent years, the practical application of this means of identification has become increasingly important. Active research is going on to attempt to answer the question of just how unique is a person's voice or manner of speaking. Is an individual's voice a unique, relatively fixed, and unchanging biological characteristic which is distinctive enough to identify him as are key biological features including fingerprints, blood groups, etc.?

The Biology of Vocalizations

Phonetics is the science of speech sounds and their production. It includes the study of the way sounds are formed by the organs of speech and the way sounds affect the organs of hearing. The remarkable studies being done with language communication in chimpanzees notwithstanding, no other animal has come close to the spectacular achievement of man in the development of speech. One may be amazed at the diversity of languages and the sounds that are emphasized and utilized by different peoples throughout the world. Although at times it may appear that there is no way the same human physical structures could be used to produce such diverse sounds, it is true, nevertheless, that all spoken languages make use of the same organs of speech. Some languages, including English, make use largely of vowels and

42

consonants. In other languages, there may be more use of gutturals, of changes in tone, and of "clicks" of the tongue.

The basic organs of speech include the lips, teeth, cheeks, jaws, tongue, palate, pharynx, larynx, and vocal cords (Fig. 10). The larynx or voice box is the most important of the vocal organs. Although it is possible to learn to speak by expelling air from the esophagus if the larynx has to be removed because of certain diseases, the quality of voice is changed drastically. Typically, sounds are generated as air leaves the lungs and passes the different speech organs. The shape of the air passages is changed by the movement of the speech organs. Our various sounds of consonants and vowels are due to the changes which the air passages undergo and which modify the air passing through them. Vowels, for example, are produced by air flowing freely through the air passages, whereas consonants are a result of the air passages being blocked, partially or completely.

Different vocal cavities act as resonators in the production of voice. The major vocal cavities are the throat, the nose, and the mouth. The resonators serve to increase the magnitude of the sound. Since the vocal cavities of all individuals are most unlike-

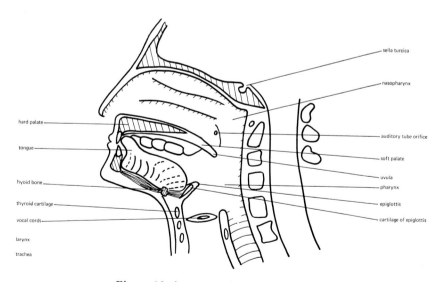

Figure 10. Anatomy of the vocal system.

ly to be identical, the likelihood that no two individuals will produce the same vocal sounds is increased. It must be realized that the voice of an individual also may be altered by sickness or by conscious effort. In the case of a sinus congestion, as in a heavy cold, one or more of the air sinuses may be blocked and the individual is told, "You sound as if you had a cold." If the infection is severe enough, it may spread to the vocal cords themselves and, if they cannot vibrate properly, the voice may be lost completely (laryngitis) or reduced to a whisper. The same condition may be achieved on the part of a sports fan who shouts himself hoarse.

Other changes in voice take place during normal aging. The high-pitched voices of children are due to differences in the anatomical structure of the speech organs. The vocal cords, resonators, and sinuses all tend to be smaller. Dramatic changes in the voice take place in males at the time of puberty. The vocal cords and the front part of the thyroid cartilage (Adam's apple) thicken and get heavier.

Physical Qualities of Sound

In order to understand the principles upon which voice identification rests, it is necessary to comment briefly about certain aspects of the physical qualities of sound, including frequency, pitch, and intensity. The human ear can distinguish two or more sounds, provided the sounds differ in one or more of the characteristics of loudness, quality, or pitch. Pitch is associated primarily with frequency. The frequency of a sound is the interval of time between each successive pulse in a sound wave. Loudness or intensity is associated with the rate at which energy is transmitted to the ear. Quality is related to the complexity of the sound waves.

The sensitivity of the human ear to the range of frequency varies considerably among different individuals. For the average normal ear, it is from 20 to 20,000 vibrations per second.

With an understanding of the physics of sound and hearing, it has been possible to devise instruments, such as the sound spectrograph, to receive and record sound waves. Lawrence Kersta, working for Bell Telephone Laboratories at the time, adapted and applied the sound spectrograph (Fig. 11) to problems of

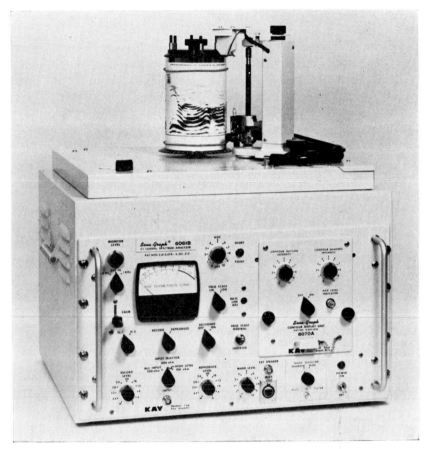

Figure 11. A sound spectrograph. Courtesy of Kay Elemetrics Corp.

personal identification. Kersta proceeded on the assumption that the pictorial representation of an individual's voice or voiceprint should be as unique as any of his other unique biological attributes.

The output of the sound spectrograph is a visual display in which a person's speech is broken down into three primary components, which are displayed on a spectrogram. Each word or phrase has a characteristic pattern on the spectrogram based on the time, frequencies, and relative amplitude. Two types of spectrograms or voiceprints are utilized in voiceprint identifica-

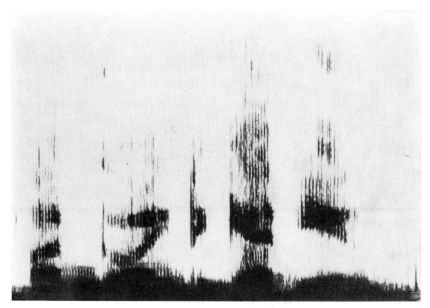

Figure 12. A bar spectrogram. The spectrograph has recorded a speaker saying, "I'm going to get you."

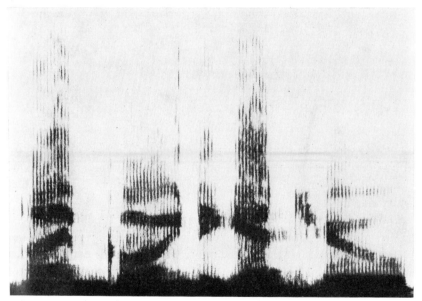

Figure 13. A bar spectrogram of a different speaker saying, "I'm going to get you."

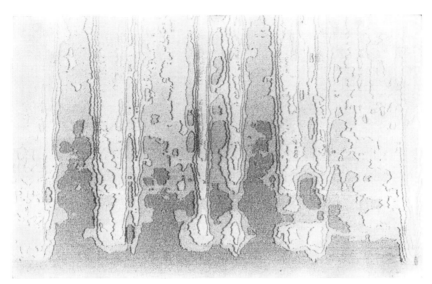

Figure 14. A contour voiceprint. This illustration is a print of the bar spectrogram which is illustrated in Figure 12.

tion. These are the bar voiceprint (Figs. 12 and 13) and the contour voiceprint (Fig. 14). In the former, resonance bars of the voice are displayed with *dimensions* of time, frequency, and loudness. In the latter, as the name implies, the *levels* of loudness, time, and frequency are displayed.

The voiceprints of each individual, according to Kersta, will be unique as a result of the uniqueness of each person's vocal apparatus, including the vocal cords and the articulators, and the way the individual has developed their usage.

If the voiceprint of a suspect matches that of an unknown voiceprint, then one might conclude that the two voiceprints were, in fact, produced by the same individual. Although the spectrograms of the same words or phrases produced by the same individual are never likely to be completely identical, there will be much more overall similarity than those spectrograms produced by two different individuals. Hence, individuals can be identified on the basis of a detailed visual examination of spectrograms. In his early studies at the Bell Research Laboratories, Kersta indicated that there was less than a 1 percent chance of a wrong identification using voiceprints.

With the great potential legal application of voice identification, legitimate questions have been raised concerning the accuracy and reliability of the method. Preliminary evaluation was accomplished by Tosi (1967, 1968), who observed an error of 6.3 percent in trials of identification. The most comprehensive testing program to date has been conducted by the Department of Audiology and Speech Sciences of Michigan State University. Details of the study have been published in a comprehensive report entitled "Voice Identification Research" (1972). In the study, twenty-nine persons received training as listeners for a period of one month. A total of 250 persons were used as speakers during the experimental trials. The speakers were randomly chosen from male students at Michigan State University. All speakers were United States natives and spoke general American English dialect with no speech defects. The speakers each recorded nine clue words at two sessions held one month apart. The clue words were common words: it – is – on – you – and – the – I – to – me. The words were spoken in isolation, in a fixed context, and in a random context. Additional experimental trials made use of six clue words. Both "open" and "closed" trials were used. In the open trials, the examiners had to decide whether the matching spectrograms were or were not produced by one of the known speakers. In addition, the known speakers had to be selected. In the closed trials, one of the known speakers always produced the spectrogram, and a correct match had to be made.

The overall results appeared quite good, and it would seem that voiceprint identification holds a great promise in its potential applications in law enforcement. The Michigan State University study concludes that the results

suggest that experienced examiners can identify or eliminate one unknown speaker from among as many as 40 known speakers, with little difference in accuracy being evidence in the use of nine or six clue words. The expected percentage of errors made by examiners who are forced to reach a positive decision in every trial of speaker identification they perform (using *exclusively* visual examination of spectrograms) varies according to the conditions involved in each type of trial.

The report continues as follows:

These findings suggest that if an experienced examiner, using only Visual Inspection of Spectrograms for legal purposes of identification and excluding any kind of listening, is forced to reach a positive decision in each case (devoting approximately 15 minutes to complete the task), his expected error range would be 14-18 percent. The probability that his wrong decisions will eliminate a guilty person is 75 percent of the total expected error. The probability that when in error this examiner will accuse an innocent person is 25 percent of the total expected error.

Under the specified conditions, the expected range of false identification is 5-6 percent and the expected range of the elimination of a guilty person is 10-12 percent.

Analysis of the ratings in the scale of self confidence used by the examiners in this project showed that approximately 60 percent of their wrong decisions were graded as "uncertain." This finding suggests that the examiners' errors could have been reduced to approximately 40 percent of the observed figure, were these examiners not forced to reach a positive decision for the trials in which they felt uncertain.

Clearly, the repeated errors apply to experimental trials in which the examiners used visual inspection of spectrograms exclusively, devoting an average of fifteen minutes per trial in reaching a forced positive decision. It could be hypothesized that if in addition to visual comparisons of spectrograms the examiners had not been forced to reach a decision when uncertain and had been allowed to listen to the unknown and known voices, the errors might have been further reduced. The experiment performed by Stevens et al. (1968), as well as the opinion of some phoneticians and linguists who feel that speaker recognition by listening is more accurate than by visual comparison of spectrograms, seems to confirm this hypothesis.

Practical Applications

The 1972 "Voice Identification Research" report also summarizes the results of practical cases involving the voice identification service. Since 1967, a total of 291 cases involving 27 different types of crimes were referred to the service. The results were summarized as follows.

As a result of the study of 42,432 spectrograms, 673 voices

were examined; 105 persons were identified as the unknown or questioned voice on tape recordings; 172 persons were eliminated as the unknown or questioned voice on tape recordings. For various reasons, a definite opinion could not be rendered concerning the other 396 persons. It was not always sensible to obtain information from the investigating officers that would substantiate the opinions of the voice identification examiners. However, it was reported that in thirty cases, those persons identified by voice identification techniques later made confessions or admissions correlating voice identification opinions. No information was found to prove the wrong person had been identified by voice identification techniques.

Use of Voiceprint Identification in the Courtroom

Until the publication of the Michigan State University study, voiceprint identification, with few exceptions, had not been considered admissible evidence. Gocke and Oleniewski (1973) have presented a brief historical review of the use of voiceprint identification in the courtroom. Several court cases were described in which voiceprints were utilized.

In the case of *Trimble v. Hedman* (1971), a telephone call for emergency aid led to the ambush and killing of a police officer. A voiceprint of the recording of the emergency caller was made and was later compared to voiceprints taken from suspects of the killing. Comparison of the voiceprints indicated that the anonymous voiceprint belonged to the defendant, Trimble. The Minnesota Supreme Court, however, would not permit voiceprints to be the sole means of identifying a suspected criminal.

In the second case described by Gocke and Oleniewski, *United States v. Raymond,* voiceprints were used to match the defendant with the voice of an unknown caller. Judge Oliver Gasch accepted the evidence stating, "It is on the basis of the extensive Tosi study, his testimony in open court, and the opinions expressed by other experts, that this court concludes spectrogram analysis is admissible evidence."

Education and Training

It is obvious that, as in other branches of forensic science, both formal education and considerable training are necessary in order to become an expert examiner in voiceprint identification. The Michigan State University School of Criminal Justice has made the following recommendations with regard to training and educational requisites:

1. Ideally, the voiceprint identification expert should hold a baccalaureate degree in either speech science or physical science.
2. While it has been demonstrated that acceptable second-generation trainees can be recruited from a general population, law enforcement technicians with comparative identification expertise are the recommended trainees.
3. In the absence of a baccalaureate degree as suggested above, the following college-level courses are strongly urged as a prerequisite to eventual use of the voiceprint identification technique: phonetics, acoustics (with the accompanying basic physics), speech science, linguistics, audiology, and basic electronics.
4. Thorough training in the preparation of tape recordings and voice spectrograms is necessary.
5. Enrollment in a carefully supervised training program in voice spectrogram identification should be required until the trainee reaches a 99 percent level of accuracy in closed trials working with spectrograms made from a homogeneous population.
6. Upon satisfactory completion of a training program similar to what has been outlined above, the trainee should then undergo apprenticeship instruction with an experienced supervisor.

Although it is one of the newest fields in forensic science, voiceprint identification has a definite, albeit somewhat restricted, usefulness in the crime laboratory. The laboratory studies and the actual cases involving this means of individual identification have been found to yield an accuracy and reliability similar to those observed with most other types of individual identification.

CHAPTER 5

Personal Appearance Identification

PERSONAL APPEARANCE identification is the verbal or pictorial physical description or appearance of an individual. This physical description is of great importance in the field of law enforcement, as it is often the only means by which the police can search for a suspected felon. In some crimes, such as assault or robbery, eyewitnesses can provide all the facts necessary for the apprehension of the criminal.

The development of the first modern system of identification is attributed to Alphonse M. Bertillon, working for the Paris Police in the Identification Section in 1882. Prior to that time, criminal identification was accomplished by detectives who would attend lineups of criminals and try to memorize faces for future recognition if the criminal were to be later involved in another crime. Photography was only beginning to be used to record the faces of convicts.

Bertillon's system proved to be a big step forward in the identification process. His method included both full-face and profile photographs, a detailed written description, and a collection of body measurements, termed anthropometry. As each criminal was brought in, he was photographed, measured, and described, and the data were then catalogued. Although Bertillon's methods have proved themselves to be fairly accurate, they still did not provide a unique means of identifying an individual. Soon thereafter, fingerprinting came into use as a means of unique identification.

Although fingerprinting is the most absolute means of identification presently in use, personal appearance identification is the most common way to identify an individual and can often be the only means of tying a suspect to a particular crime, particularly in the early stages. Currently, four methods of personal appearance identification are used. These are (1) the "mug shot" or police photograph, (2) the artist's drawing, (3) composite kits, and (4) the verbal description or *portrait parle.* These will be discussed in greater detail later.

The Witness

In order for police agencies to obtain a victim's or witness's help successfully in a criminal's identification, the process involved in the recognition or identification of a suspect must be understood.

Many factors are capable of influencing the ability of a witness to identify or describe a suspect. These include (1) psychological factors such as stress and fear, (2) the motivation of the witness to identify a suspect, (3) the attention that was originally given to the suspect and any distractions that might have been present (such as noise), (4) the length of time elapsed since the original viewing to the identification through mug shots or a line-up and what occurred during that time, (5) the knowledge that an identification will later be made, and (6) whether or not the suspect could be seen clearly and, naturally, whether or not the suspect wore a disguise.

The witness, especially if he is also the victim, can be under stress or shock and undergo selective amnesia for those events that occurred immediately prior to the actual crime (Leonard and Zavala, 1964).

The witness's relationship with law enforcement officers can greatly influence the ability of the eyewitness to identify the suspect. This can work both to the officer's advantage and disadvantage. The witness may either be willing to cooperate with the police to the extent that he gives false information which he thinks the police want to hear, or he can be unwilling to help the police to the extent that he will either tell them nothing at all or tell them a complete falsehood.

The original attention given to the suspect is also important to the determination of identity. Longer exposure causes better memory, particularly if the witness knows in advance he is going to be making an identification and when, in addition, the file of suspects to be looked at does not number more than fifty (Alexander, 1972, and Zavala and Paley, 1972).

The time lapse between the original observation of a suspect and the viewing of him in a mug shot file or in a lineup also affects the likelihood of a correct identification. From the time that an event is first witnessed to the time that the event has to be told to someone else or an identification needs to be made, the memory of the event will decline and change (Postman and Egan, 1949).

The strength of a memory image deteriorates with the amount of items viewed after the original observation of an event (Wickelgren and Norman, 1966). The identification of a person is therefore best when done after viewing as few other faces as possible. As the number of faces seen increases, the likelihood of a correct identification diminishes (Alexander, 1972).

One way to ensure that the witness views a minimum of faces is to screen the mug shots for the witness (have the mug shots filed by offense or any other divisions that would weed out the irrelevant faces). Another method that helps in the identification process when many faces must be viewed is to allow for frequent rest breaks for the witness.

If an individual knows that he will later have to try to identify a person, his chances of success will increase (Zavala and Paley, 1972). It must be remembered, however, that the layman who has just witnessed a crime or has been the victim is not skilled in the observation skills necessary to a good identification and will often give descriptions in generalities. "He looked 'average,' with a medium build and medium height. He had no outstanding characteristics. He was just your 'average' man."

It is obvious that such a description is of little or no use, and with such descriptions it is very difficult to obtain a definite picture of an individual.

It must also be remembered that anyone who witnesses a crime usually does so involuntarily and without forewarning. The witness is therefore not ready for what he observes and is often scared or startled. Because of the shock, the details of the event may not be incorporated into the memory or may be remembered only partially.

Another factor which influences the ability of a witness to identify a suspect is the type and quality of the mug shots.

Statistically, there is no single best pose position for facial identification (Lane, 1972).

It should be noted that as the number of photographs of any one person increases, so does the percentage of correct identifications. It is therefore best to have as a minimum a front and a profile shot on file. The use of color film instead of black and white, and the use of video tape or movie sequences of either black and white or color also improves the identification success rate (Zavala and Paley, 1972).

Concerning the sex of the witness, it has been found that in adults, there is no substantial difference in the identification success rates of men and women (Howells, 1938; Strong, 1912; Lieberman and Culpepper, 1965).

As far as the actual physical characteristics are concerned, those features which are most frequently cited by subjects who have proven themselves to be good identifiers in research are facial markings (moles, beauty marks, freckles, etc.), eye color, and teeth (Zavala and Paley, 1972).

Interviewing the Witness

As opposed to fingerprints or voiceprints, which are obtained firsthand by the investigator, personal appearance identification is usually secondhand information obtained through a witness' description. The weakness of personal appearance identification is that it is only as reliable as the witness. A witness can be anyone and hence have any sort of character.

When considering the reliability of a witness, the investigating officer must take into account whether or not the witness is of a weak character and subject to influence, coercion, or intimidation. He must also consider whether or not the witness is credible. Would the witness's vision and the night darkness have allowed him to see what he claims he saw?

Eyewitnesses should, in addition, be able to account for their presence at the scene of the crime or of their acquaintance with the suspect or victim. The witness's history as a witness and his criminal involvement record should also be checked to help determine his reliability.

To be effective, the interviewers should question the witness as soon as possible, as time reduces memory. Prior to the interview, the witness should not be allowed to listen to or discuss the case with any other witnesses, as this can cause the witness to change his statement. The interviewer must also take care to ask the relevant questions in such a way that they do not lead the witness in a direction favorable to the officer or antagonize the witness so that he gives an unfavorable description. In this respect, the relationship between the officer and the witness will help to determine the results of the interview.

The interviewing officer should try to win the confidence of the witness with a positive attitude from the onset of their meeting; he should also try to be as friendly and as relaxed as possible. The best interview is one in which the witness voluntarily divulges his complete information. To force a description from a witness can alter the reliability of the information. Questions should be made easy to understand, and the interviewer should let the witness describe the event in his own way.

The interviewing officer must be extremely careful about his choice of words and should know the suggestibility that words can have. Probably a fair number of those witnesses who have falsely accused people were led to their descriptions by interviewers who unknowingly implied the answers that they sought. Witnesses have been known to change their stories or identify someone they have never even seen because of the way an interviewer has unintentionally worded a question (Loftus, 1974).

With a little bit of care and forethought, however, the interviewer should be able to overcome many of the flaws commonly associated with personal appearance identification and obtain a reliable description.

Criminal Photographs (Mug Shots)

Recent photographs are the most accurate means of personal appearance identification, as they provide the best likeness of an individual. The problems with mug shots are that only photographs of known and local felons are readily available to the law enforcement officer. Still, with the initiation of the camera into the law enforcement field, the accuracy of personal appearance identification took a great step forward.

At the present time, mug shots usually consist of two photographs—a full-face shot and a profile shot. They are usually stored in books or files and are most frequently classified according to offense.

As to classifying types of photographs according to their worth, pictures of any sort are more valuable than descriptions. Color photographs are better than black and white (the extra detail that the color gives can be beneficial in determining identity). Better yet are video sequences that allow a witness to observe the actual movements of known felons.

In addition to video files of felons, the future trend of mug shots appears to be computerization. It probably will not be long before photographs of all known felons will be entered into a centralized crime computer, allowing an agency to draw on the mug shots of all other agencies to help in the identification of a suspect.

The Artist's Drawing

As in any other type of personal appearance identification, the artist's drawing or the composite can be no better than the witness's description. If the witness's description of a suspect is poor, there is no way possible for a good drawing to result. It is not easy to produce a successful drawing from description alone.

In addition, the process of drawing a picture of a suspect from description alone is a time-consuming task for which it is difficult to find skilled artists. It is possible, however, to achieve excellent results when a witness with a good description and a skilled artist work together.

The two methods used by police artists are one in which the artist works with the witnesses to produce an individually described drawing and another in which the final drawing is a composite of the descriptions given by the witnesses. Both techniques involve a trial-and-error method by which a witness will tell the artist what a feature looked like, the artist will then try to draw it, and the witness will make corrections. In both methods, when more than one witness is present, they should be initially separated and prevented from discussing the event so that they will retain their initial impressions.

The Police Artist in Action

The following account is provided by Craig Pursley, a consultant artist for the Fort Collins, Colorado, Police Department. His description of his activities provides an excellent look at the actual operations of a police artist:

> The standard television image of a police artist is usually not a true one. They generally show the witness finalizing his description by saying something like, "The nose needs to be a little wider." The change is made, and the witness says, "That's him!" And it is! It almost always looks just like the suspect. This is usually not the case in actual police drawing. It is not because the artist does not have the ability, but rather the witness does not generally have that good a memory.
>
> Most of the cases end with the witness saying, "that's not quite right, but I do not know why. . . ." Remembering is the biggest hurdle to the drawing. In fact, it was shown in one study that a witness forgets about 90 percent of the description in the first twenty-four hours. Unless there was some outstanding or unusual feature, the witness may remember only hair length and color and sometimes the facial shape.
>
> But let me start where I begin the drawing. First, I have the victim or witness look through the mug shots, not for the actual suspect but for someone with similar characteristics such as hair, facial shape, eyes, and so on. Once the photos with general similarities are withdrawn from the file (sometimes as many as six mug shots), I assemble the parts into one drawing. When the line drawing is completed, I let the witness take a good look at it and make the changes he feels are necessary. Once that is finished to his satisfaction, the shading is added. The latter shows hollowness or fullness of cheeks, deep-set eyes, protruding forehead, crooked nose, complexion, age, etc.
>
> Usually, the more changes the witness makes, the better his memory. Most often, the drawing takes about ninety minutes.
>
> One drawing of a rape suspect took four hours, and when the suspect was arrested four days later, it proved the witness's good memory. The next drawing, however, of a sexual assault suspect, was not so good. It took only fifteen minutes from start to finish. The victim made no changes in the drawing. The suspect is still at large.
>
> Other factors enter into the success of the drawing besides the artwork and the memory of the witness. One is a relaxed atmosphere. Another is separation of witnesses, if there are more than one. Too often when witnesses are together they disagree and confuse each other. Ei-

ther do one drawing from the witness who got the best look at the suspect or do two different drawings.

By far the most challenging drawing I have done was of a very unusual nature. It was a murder case with no witnesses and an unidentified victim. He had a broken jaw, broken nose, shattered cheekbone, and cuts and bruises all over his face. In order to help identify the victim, I had to go to the morgue and draw what I felt the victim must have looked like before the homicide. I do not know how close I came to his former appearance, but I am sure the hour and a half spent drawing a battered murder victim was the strangest ninety minutes of my life.

Example of a "Case Study"

In order to gain a better perspective of the police artist at work, it was decided to create an example. Although the example obviously is artificial, it does serve to illustrate the procedure and the problems that may arise.

In this case, two "victims" were placed together in a room. A person, whom they had never seen before, entered the room and spent two minutes chatting with the "victims." Both victims knew in advance that they would be describing the suspect to a police artist. One victim was a college student with an interest in law enforcement, and the other victim was a professional silversmith. The victims in this example thus probably represent persons more accustomed to using their powers of observation than the average victim. They also were able to make their observations unclouded by any other emotional factors.

After the two-minute session with the suspect ended, one victim joined the artist in another room for the first drawing. The first session lasted approximately one hour. After the first drawing was completed, the first victim left the room and the second victim went through a similar procedure with the artist. It should also be noted that the police artist had never seen the suspect before and that there were no prior mug shots in the files.

Results of the two drawings and an actual photograph of the suspect are shown in Figure 15. It is evident that neither drawing matches up exactly with the photograph. It also is evident that both drawings contain some good features.

The work of the police artist is one more link in the chain of

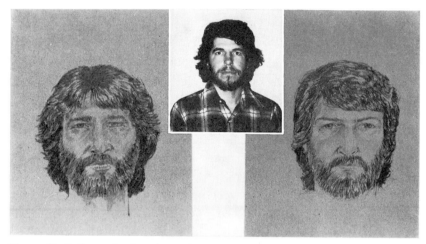

Figure 15. Police artist drawings of a "suspect" based on separate descriptions of two different eyewitnesses and an actual photograph of the "suspect."

identification procedures, and at times it can be remarkably effective.

The Composite

To help reduce the problems of not always having a skilled police artist available, commercial composites were developed. These kits allow anyone trained in their use to produce a reasonable general appearance of a suspect (provided the witness has a good description), although they do not allow the fine detail possible in an artist's drawing.

Two major types currently available on a commercial basis are *Identi-kit* and *Photo-fit®*. The kits are pictures of different facial features, either drawn or photographic, that are pieced together to make a complete face. Human faces can be reduced to a small number of parts, with a relatively small number of types of each part which can, in turn, be combined to make a practically endless variety of composite combinations.

The first type of commercial composite is the *Identi-kit*. This is a series of transparencies with drawings of eyes, noses, hair, mustaches and beards, age lines, glasses, headgear, and lips. The witness decides which transparency of each feature most closely resembles the suspect, and the transparencies are then fit together. Finer details can be added with a grease pencil.

In order to improve the faults of *Identi-kit,* identification kits using photographs rather than drawings were developed. One of these, *Photo-fit,* starts with general face outlines (angular or round) and then adds the features. Another method of using photographs in identification is for a department to maintain its own file of general photographs of features for a witness to look at when trying to describe a suspect.

Portrait Parle

Portrait parle is the verbal description of someone and is most effective when used in conjunction with a mug shot or drawing. The following *portrait parle* is a fairly detailed one that should allow for most of the information that a law enforcement officer would need to know. The most effective method of making a verbal description is to start at the top of the body and work down, and to start with a general description and move to specifics.

Full Description of an Individual (Allison, 1973)

Name (full): alias, nickname.
Date of Birth:
Present and Former Address:
Nationality:
Social Security Number:
Military Serial Number:
Fingerprint Classification:
Sex: (Could it have been a flat-chested female or a male with feminine characteristics?)
Height:
Weight:
Build: Stocky, thin, medium, fat, muscular.
Age: (Did the suspect look older or younger than he actually was? Why? Did he seem mature and sure of himself?)
Race:

General Impression: Type; personality; social status; did he remind the witness of someone else? Who? Why?

Scars, Marks, Tattoos: Type, color, size, location.

General Appearance: Any nervous mannerisms, conditions.

Head: Shape (round, square, triangular, oval, flat on top, flat in back, thin, long, short, bulgy in back, high on top).

Face: Expression (innocent look, happy or sad appearance), age lines, fullness, size deformities, positions of features.

Complexion: Color (fair, sunburnt, ruddy, pale), freckled, texture (oily, acne, pock marked, dry, smooth), moles, beauty marks.

Forehead: Slope (vertical, receding, medium, prominent, bulgy), width (narrow, medium, wide), heavily wrinkled, high or low forehead.

Hairline: Baldness (total, total receding, receding over temple, frontal, frontal and occipital, entire top of head), widow's peak.

Hair: Color (white, gray, salt and pepper, blonde, brown, red, black). Does it look dyed (different colored roots, streaked, frosted)? Length (crew cut, short, at ears, below ears, collar length, etc.), location of part (right side, left side, middle, none), texture (straight, wavy, curly, kinky, wiry, fine, normal, thick), quantity (thin, normal, thick, balding), style (shagged, crew cut, normal, neat, messy), use of hair spray or dressing.

Headgear: Did he wear hat or mask? Style, texture, kind.

Eyebrows: Color, type (heavy, thin, absent, bushy), shape (slanting upward or downward, straight, arched, long, short, narrow, wide), penciled, plucked.

Glasses: Shape, wire or plastic rimmed, tinted lenses, color of frames, size, thickness of lens, bifocal, half-moon, contact lenses.

Eyes: Color (blue, gray, green, hazel, brown, black, pink), eyelashes (length, thickness, mascara), eyelids (wrinkled, puffy), size (small, medium, large), shape (wide, narrow, slanted toward nasal or temple side, rounded), makeup (eyeliner, eye shadow, color, amount), expression (serious eyes, relaxed, penetrating), pupils (size), position in socket (normal, protruding, deep-set, sunken), distance between (close-set, wide-set, normal), abnormalities (nervous condition, squinting, excess blinking, missing eye, glass eye, watery, bloodshot, crossed).

Cheeks: Coloring, dimples, structure (high cheekbones, sunken, full, thin, normal, jowls), makeup.

Ears: Size (small, medium, large), earrings (pierced, normal, post, dangling, more than one hole per ear, location of hole), shape (square, rectangular, round, oval), position on head (high, low, normal), set to head (close-set, normal, protruding from head), earlobe (size, pointed, rounded, square, attached to head or not), patterns of inner ear.

Nose: Bridge (flat, small, medium, large), width (narrow, medium, wide), projection (long, medium, short), distance between nose and mouth (wide, medium, narrow), length (long, medium, narrow), line (convex, concave, hooked, aquiline), tip of nose (turned-up, turned-down, horizontal, rounded, pointed), nostrils (showing, hidden, flared, small), deformities.

Facial Hair: Length (unshaven, few days growth, short, medium, long), color, type (mustache, beard, sideburns, clean shaven), style (beard—pointed, square-cut, rounded, goatee, etc.; mustache—short, combed to side, combed down, handlebar, etc.; sideburns—close-cut, short, long, mutton-chop), care (neat, unkempt, trimmed), quantity (thick, thin, medium, sparse, bushy).

Mouth: Lips (thin, medium, thick), lip position (normal, lower protruding, upper protruding), comparison upper and lower lips (width, length), lipstick (color, amount), expression (smile, drooping, sneer, lips compressed, corners up, one corner higher than the other, corners down), oddities, deformities, odor of breath.

Teeth: Did they show? Color (white, yellow, stained), size (long, broad, short, narrow, normal), position (normal, protruding, underbite, gaps, crowded), condition (good, decayed, broken, missing, crooked, replaced, braces).

Chin: Type (normal, receding, jutting, double-chinned), shape (pointed, full, square, round), size (small, medium, large), traits (dimpled, cleft).

Neck: Length (short, very short, medium, long), size (thick, thin, medium, very thick), marks, scars, oddities (large Adam's apple).

Body Hair: Location, amount, color.

Shoulders: Size (broad, medium, narrow), shoulder carriage (one higher than other, flat, rounded, hump-backed, drooping).

Chest: Size (narrow, broad, normal), shape (normal, deep, narrow, flat, pigeon-chested), presence of hair.

Abdomen: Shape (flat, sunken, bulging under ribs, bulging low, rounded, sagging).

Hips and Waist: Size (broad, medium, narrow), waist length (normal, long, short), seat (flat, protruding, muscle, fat).

Arms: Girth (thin, medium, large, fat, muscle), length (long, medium, short).

Hands: Width (narrow, medium, broad), length (short, medium, long), fingers (deformed, missing, short, medium, long, width, rings), fingernails (deformed, missing, short, bitten, long, normal, polished, color, dirty, clean), abnormal conditions (arthritis, extra fingers).

Legs: Length (normal, long, short, unequal), girth (thin, thick, medium, muscular, fat), shape (knock-kneed, bow-legged, normal), abnormalities (missing leg).

Feet: Size (short, medium, long), width (thin, medium, wide), abnormal conditions (pigeon-toed, flat-footed, toes turned out).

Speech: Accent, educated-sounding, slurred, volume (loud or soft spoken), repeated phrases or words, pitch (high, low, squeaky, profanity, lisp, stuttering.

Dress: Type of clothes (work, business suits, sports clothes, uniform), care (well kept, little care, dirty, messy), style (old-fashioned, conservative, modern, trend-setting, flashy), jewelry (style, where worn, real or costume), footwear (shoes, boots, tennis shoes, polished, worn).

Carriage: Head (erect, held to side, held to front or back), arms (held tightly or loosely at sides, pronounced walking arm movements), hips (aligned with body, lateral movement), walk (feet slapped to the ground, tiptoe, shuffled, limped, high steps).

Friends, Associates: People works with regularly, loner, "picks up" friends, associates with criminals or noncriminals, where he "hangs out."

Usual Type of Crime: Arson, assault, fraud, murder, burglary, robbery, drugs, smuggling, kidnapping, extortion, terrorism, youth gang activity, etc. (describe type of crime and modus operandi).

Weapons: Type normally carries or has been known to carry, skilled at hand-to-hand combat, razor, knife (type), sap or blackjack, brass knuckles, firearms (make, caliber, barrel length), rifle, shotgun, revolver, semi-automatic, others, number of weapons carried? Where carried? Location of gun (pocket, belt holster, right or left handed, regular or cross draw, shoulder holster, tucked in pants waist, wrist, ankle or groin holster, holster at top of coat sleeve, in hat). Does he use the weapon? What for? Is it just to threaten or intimidate?

Tobacco: Chewing, snuff, or smoking tobacco. Brand used. Does he smoke cigarettes, cigars, or a pipe?

Alcohol: Type of drinker (social, solitary, heavy or moderate drinker), type of alcohol and brand (beer, whisky, wine, vodka, gin, rum), location of drinking (bars, at home, cocktail lounges), drinking conduct (quiet, depressed, aggressive, boisterous, drowsy, crying).

Eating Habits: Type of food, where eats.

Sexual Habits: Heterosexual (single partner, bar pickups, street pickups, call girls, likes and dislikes), homosexual.

Other specific habits, traits, or perversions.

Obviously, the way the *portrait parle* is handled is going to be different for known and unknown felons, although it should be as thorough as possible for both types.

In summary, the best method of personal appearance identification is a recent photograph, followed by an artist's drawing, a composite, and lastly, a well-prepared verbal description (which can be very effective in the hands of a trained officer).

These methods of identification should be used in varying degrees, depending upon the circumstances. A brief, general verbal description, including a clothing description, will be used to air over the police radio if a crime has just occurred. A more in-depth description with pictures should be used in the squad room, and the greatest detail, including the *portrait parle,* should be available to those responsible for the follow-up.

Although personal appearance identification is the oldest method of human identification in existence, it is by no means outdated and will continue to be a very valuable asset to law enforcement.

CHAPTER 6

Forensic Anthropology

MICHAEL CHARNEY

Introduction

THE QUESTION sometimes arises, "Who was this passel of bones when it graced a living person?" Skeletons of humans are constantly being found in all sorts of places; behind a clump of bushes by a pair of would-be lovers, in a desert by a "desert rat," fished from a river by a fisherman, and, yes, even in closets and attics. Sometimes a skull shows evidence of violence such as a great gash or jagged hole, such as one found in an Oklahoma City attic by a new female tenant.

The identification of human remains is the responsibility of the local law enforcement agency where such remains are found. Human bodies whose flesh is so necrotic, so decomposed that the usual signs of sex are missing must then be reduced to bone for study. Some physical anthropologists are trained in human morphology and osteology to prepare them for research in human evolution and the biological classification of human races. It is to these scientists that the police will turn for aid in expert analysis of human remains.

Law enforcement agencies will seek the services of experts in many fields, for it would be too much to expect the individual police officer to be all-knowing in all areas that are peripheral to his work.

It was an axiom of the buccaneers who plundered ships on the Spanish mains and all other sea lanes, that "dead men tell no tales." And so, the prisoner walks the plank with securely tied hands to a watery grave. Professor of Anthropology J. E. Pearce wrote a treatise entitled "Tales That Dead Men Tell" (1935). Professor Pearce was absorbed in the cultural remains that archaeology uncovers and studies giving insight as to the lifestyles of dead societies. Physically, dead men also tell tales of who they might have been when alive; their race, sex, stature, age at time of death, and any pathological condition evidenced by bones, such as arthritis and the like. Sometimes, because of some group concept of beauty, changes in skull slope brought about deliberately, such as flattening of one portion of the skull or other, can even pinpoint the tribal identity.

All this kind of information can be vital in the individual identification of a "passel of bones," and so, one more name can be struck from the Missing Persons File.

General Considerations

To be able to identify human bones as to race, sex, age at time of death, and all other such information, it is first imperative that one be thoroughly familiar with the individual bones of the human skeleton. It is not enough to recognize these bones in the unbroken state, but one must be able to do so when faced with a fragment. Providing a landmark or two are present, such fragments are no obstacle to the trained. There is no substitute for careful and thorough study for the would-be professional in this or any other field of knowledge.

This is not meant to discourage the law enforcement officer from preliminary study of bones. He can acquire a good working knowledge of the aspects of human bones and arrive at a tentative diagnosis. However, it should only be tentative. There are twenty-eight physical anthropologists, expert in this work, dispersed throughout the country, who are members of the Physical Anthropology section of the American Academy of Forensic Scientists. Their services are at the command of law enforcement agencies.

For the working police officer who would like to gain more knowledge in this area, I can recommend several books, laboratory manuals, and the like for study. This chapter, for one, will summarize the details of sexing, racing, and aging bones. This information is also available in Charney (1974), Krogman (1962), Olivier (1969), and Singh and Bhasin (1968). For material on individual bone study and interpretations, there are Charney (1974), Bass (1971), Brothwell (1972), and the standard textbooks of anatomy, both descriptive and functional.

An important aspect of bone identification is being able to assign laterality, that is right or left side. I once received a burial from the archaeology students at the then Boise State College. This one burial contained two bones of the upper arm; all normal people have two such bones. However, they were both from the right side! We had here the elements of at least two individuals.

You can readily see that the ability to tell to which side of the body a bone belongs is imperative.

Is It Human Or?

The first consideration is to know whether the bones in question are human or of some other animal.

You might think that a decision as to human or animal is not particularly difficult. This is true if you have the skull, but other bones are not that simple if you are without knowledge in this field. It is uncanny how the hands and feet of the bear, especially cubs, will trick you into thinking they are human. Hunters will skin a bear, then saw off the paws to be left behind. I have had two such feet submitted for analysis by sheriffs of Colorado counties. For a discussion of this, see Charney (1974), and Stewart (1959).

Man, that is *Homo sapiens,* is an annoyingly variable creature, as is all living matter. Hence, the following descriptions are not to be taken as all-or-none features of the sexes and races. The traits that delineate sex, race, age, and so forth will apply generally, though not in every single individual. If given enough bones of a person, you should be able to carry through to victory in the majority of cases.

Sexing Criteria

The determination of sex provides little problem in the living, fully clothed of course. It is certainly no problem when examining the nude body. Regardless of outer appearances, the trained eye can tell the sex of an individual at a glance and be right at least 95 percent of the time. A woman's hips, for example, are a reflection of the skeletal structure underneath them—the pelvic bones comprising the innominates, the sacrum, and the coccygeal bones. In general, the woman has narrow shoulders and wide

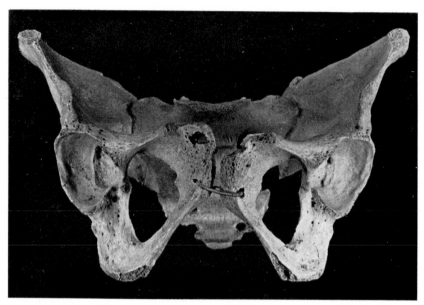

Figure 16. Pelvis from a human female. Note that the iliac bones are under-splayed. Photograph by Mark Riedo.

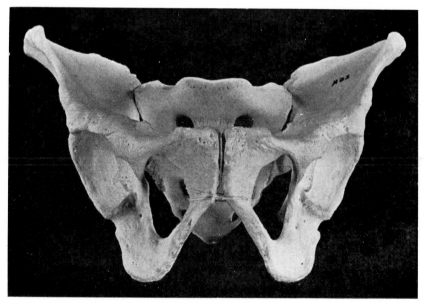

Figure 17. Pelvis from a human male.

hips, relative to the man's wide shoulders and narrow hips. Most women, because of this structuring, cannot suspend their arms straight down as does the soldier at attention; their arms must clear the hips and so angle a bit. Figures 16 and 17 show the body structure of the pelvis of male and female. You can see at a glance the undersplayed iliac bones of the female (the bones of the upper innominate) which can house the developing fetus. The very fact of sexual dimorphism, of having two separate sexes, with one sex carrying the responsibility of childbearing, has, in man, made for the important anatomical differences one readily sees in the pelvic bones. The bones of the pelvis, when available for study, will enable the expert to quickly and easily determine the sex in 95 percent of cases.

The innominate, taken feature by feature, is described in the following sections.

THE SUBPUBIC ANGLE. This is the angle made by the lower borders of the pubic bones when in opposition or contact (Fig. 18). It can be taken on one pubis only. One need only double the angle found.

To determine the angle, draw a straight line on a clean sheet of paper. Place the bone on the paper so that the pubic face touches and is parallel to this line. Now, with your pencil, run

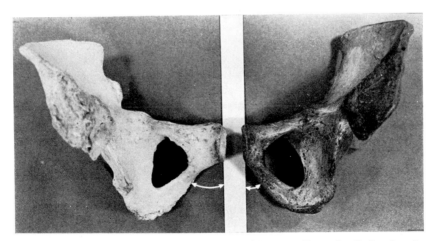

Figure 18. Subpubic angle. Right: male, with a small angle. Left: female, with a large angle.

along the edge of the bone as it curves away from the base of the pubic face. With a protracter set along the straight line, determine the angle subtended.

An angle of 90 degrees or over is indicative of female. The angle for a male will be less than 90 degrees.

ANGLE OF THE GREATER SCIATIC NOTCH. This is the deep indentation of the rear of the innominate where the ischial portion joins the ilium, above the deep pocket that takes the head of the femur, or thigh bone (Figs. 19 and 20). To measure this angle, place the bone on a sheet of clean paper, and with a pencil trace the margins of the notch. With a straight edge, draw straight lines tangential to the irregular lines traced. Place the protracter at 0-180 on one of the two lines and read off the angle made by the second line. An angle over 68 degrees is generally female, less than 68 degrees is male.

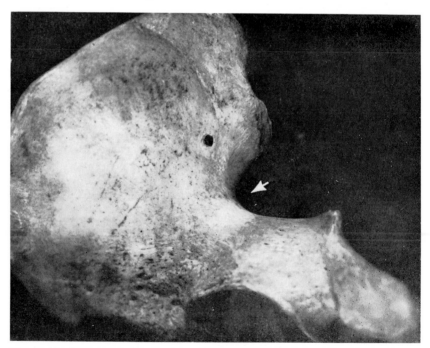

Figure 19. Greater sciatic notch of the iliac bone in the male. The notch is deep and narrow. From Charles G. Wilber, *Forensic Biology for the Law Enforcement Officer,* 1974. Courtesy of Charles C Thomas, Publisher, Springfield, Illinois.

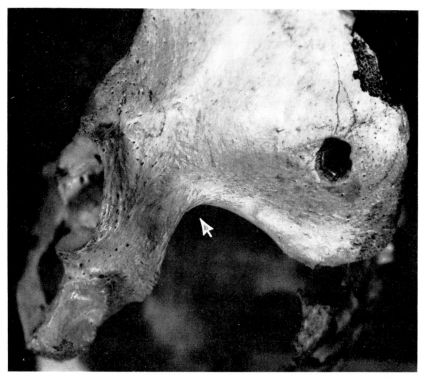

Figure 20. Greater sciatic notch for the iliac bone in the female. The notch is shallow and wide. From Charles G. Wilber, *Forensic Biology for the Law Enforcement Officer,* 1974. Courtesy of Charles C Thomas, Publisher, Springfield, Illinois.

OTHER CRITERIA FOR SEXING THE PELVIC BONES. The length (depth) of the pubic symphysis is greater in males. The acetabulum is larger in males. The obdurator foramen is larger and generally oval shaped in males. It is smaller and more triangular in females. The female sacrum is straight when compared to that of the male. A groove, the preauricular surface, when present is consistent with the female specimen (Fig. 21). A technique for sexing measures the length of the ischium and pubis from a fixed point on the acetabulum. This method is a bit tricky and best left to the experts.

The sexing of pelvis in the preadolescent and child has always been a difficulty, to the point where it is rarely attempted. The

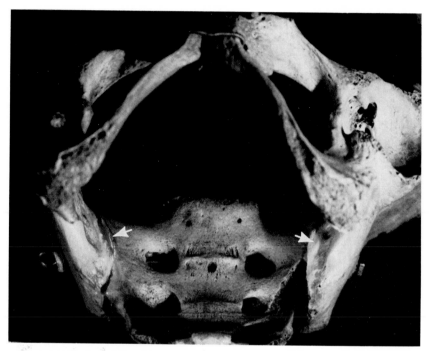

Figure 21. Sexual Dimorphism: Preauricular sulcus, female. Arrows point to sulci on each innominate bone. View is from the bottom looking through the pelvic outlet. From Charles G. Wilber, *Forensic Biology for the Law Enforcement Officer,* 1974. Courtesy of Charles C Thomas, Publisher, Springfield, Illinois.

following workers believe some diagnosis as to sex is possible in the nonadult: Thomson (1899), Reynolds (1945, 1947), Imbrie and Wyburn (1958).

The Skull as a Sex Object?

Bass (1971) and others state that the skull is probably second-best when it comes to sexing. Comas (1960) warns that it takes constant, careful practice with the skull to arrive at an accuracy of 90 percent in sexing. It is important at the outset to warn the student to compare only skulls within the particular breeding population. Some human groups are taller, heavier, and more robust than others. It is easy to see that a female skull of just such a robust population, such as the Australian aborigines, would be mistaken for a male, especially if compared to the males of many Indian (of India) groups.

Adhering religiously to these precautions, what then does one look for?

The observable differences between male and female are as follows:

1. The mastoid process is larger in males, quite small in females (Fig. 22).
2. The frontal bone is globular in females and lower vaulting in males.
3. The upper border of the eye orbit is rounded in males, sharp in females.
4. Well-developed brow ridges when present mark the male. Females for the most part lack this trait.
5. A bony occipital protuberance indicates a male. Females lack this feature (Fig. 23).
6. The posterior portion of the zygomatic process, the rear of

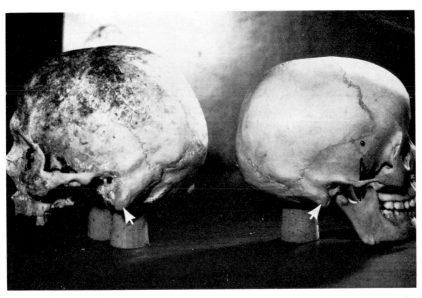

Figure 22. Sexual Dimorphism: Arrows point to large mastoid process on the male (left) and small mastoid process on the female (right). From Charles G. Wilber, *Forensic Biology for the Law Enforcement Officer,* 1974. Courtesy of Charles C Thomas, Publisher, Springfield, Illinois.

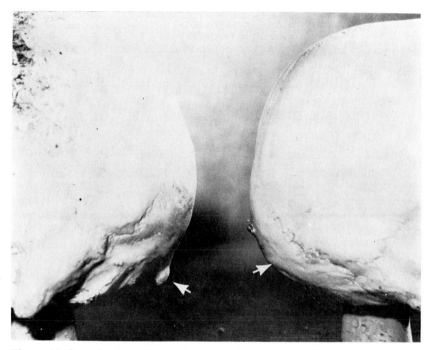

Figure 23. Sexual Dimorphism: Arrows point to extremely large external occipital protuberance on rear of male skull (left) and the absence of the protuberance on female skull (right). From Charles G. Wilber, *Forensic Biology for the Law Enforcement Officer,* 1974. Courtesy of Charles C Thomas, Publisher, Springfield, Illinois.

the curving arch of the cheek in males, extends as a ridge over and beyond the external auditory meatus, the opening to the inner ear. Unfortunately, females often show this feature.

7. In general, the male skull is larger, heavier, more robustly marked, with teeth more prominent, palate larger, mandible more robust.

The Long Bones and Others

These present problems in sexing. The long bones of the male are generally more robust, with stronger markings on the bone for muscle attachment. Hrdlicka (1952), Stewart (1959), and Pons (1955) say that the femur is the most readily sexed of all the long bones. A big head, robust neck, large condyles, and well-defined linea aspera denote the male.

The breastbone, the sternum, frequently indicates which sex in the relative lengths of the top (manubrium) to the bottom (body) portions. In males, the body will be at least twice the length of the manubrium. Females have shorter bodies.

To sum up, remember that in almost all animal and human breeding populations, females are smaller and lighter than the corresponding males. Nobody knows why this should be so. From an evolutionary viewpoint, it is not necessary. It is difficult to see just what this aspect of sexual dimorphism had to do with survival. Darwin wrestled with this problem and finally came to the conclusion that sex differences in size were probably due to sexual selection; that the male of the species picked the "little woman" when choosing a mate.

Race Determination

Probably no other aspect of man has as many "experts," not only fully informed but unshaken in their knowledge, than the concept of race. That large groups of people differ physically is obvious to any observer. To tell one of these "experts" that the study of race is not cut and dried, that criteria for biological classification cut across all races of man, that there are no clearcut racial markers that are the sole possession of one race, is received with skepticism. We think of blondism as a feature of northern Europeans and their descendants over the globe. The central desert of Australia has tribes of aborigines that show 100 percent blondism, and this can hardly be an artifact of English male contribution to the aboriginal gene pool. We think of sickle cell anemia as a central African trait, and yet there are frequencies of the gene responsible for this trait in Mediterranean countries that are not attributable to Negro gene flow. The buildup of extra enamel on the inside, lateral margins of the upper incisor teeth has been termed "shovel-shaped" by the late Alex Hrdlicka, Curator of Anthropology of the Smithsonian Institution and a leading figure in physical anthropology. Mongoloid peoples range close to the 100 percent level in the possession of this trait. It is at 100 percent level for the American Indians. Yet it is also found in Caucasians at about the 9 percent level and in Negroes at 12 percent. Again, we cannot invoke the evolutionary force of gene flow to account for this phenomenon.

Does this mean that racial diagnosis is so vague as to be next to impossible? Many cultural anthropologists and some physical anthropologists think so, and they declare that the range of variability within any breeding population is so great as to exceed the range between populations and that race classification is only the nonscientific, biased judgment of the great unwashed public. A "folk taxonomy" is the term used to denote racial categories.

And yet, were I to line up the 900 million Chinese, I doubt you would mistake one for a North European or a rain-forest-dwelling African. Not to confuse the outer physical features is one thing, but what about the skeletal framework? Are we all not "brothers under the skin?" That phrase was meant as an argument for moral persuasion and perhaps in a general way alludes to the fact that all mankind has a basic, similar biological design.

However, in the long history of man's evolution, various population groups found themselves in different ecological settings, and in response to the selection pressures of the environment, developed the several different responses that mark the major racial stocks of man. We find these differences, minor if you will, but nevertheless persistent and identifiable on the bones as well as the soft tissue. Our concern here is with the three major divisions of mankind, Caucasoid (white), Mongoloid (yellow), and Negroid (black).

In the western United States, the Mongoloids are represented in the main by the American Indians. Other Mongoloid groups such as Chinese, Japanese, etc., are far less numerous and generally localized in areas such as San Francisco, Los Angeles, and other cities. The universities and colleges have their sprinkling of Asian students. However, in the field of forensic anthropology, individual disaster identification, should one of the non-Amerindian types be missing, the community, the police would know about it. Negroids can present a problem in identification from bone, as there has been a goodly amount of gene flow from Caucasians. Many individuals who for sociological reasons are labeled Negro are biologically more Caucasoid than Negroid.

TABLE VI

RACIAL DIFFERENCES IN THE SKULL

Feature	Causasoid	Mongoloid	Negroid
Nasal Bones	narrow, high bridge	narrow, low bridge	broad and flat
Malar Bones and Arch	curved	at right angles	curved
Upper Incisors (inner surface)	smooth	shovel-shaped	smooth
Bony Brow Ridges	raised (males only)	faint, if at all	somewhat
Prognathism	rare	low frequency	prevalent
Inca Bone	rare	higher frequency	rare
Os Japonicum	rare	higher frequency	rare
Orbital borders	superior is anterior	inferior is anterior	superior is anterior

Racial differences in the skeleton, when they occur, are looked for on the skull and the long bones.

Table VI summarizes the more distinctive features on the skull of the three races.

The Nasal Bones

The nasal index, the width of the nasal opening multiplied by 100 and divided by the length, shows the following ranges in the three racial stocks:

Caucasoid .... up to 47.9% (Leptorrhine)
Mongoloid .... 48.0 to 52.9 (Mesorrhine)
Negroid .... 53.0 and up (Platyrrhine)

The greater value for Mongoloids is an artifact of the shorter length of the nose rather than an indication of a wider nose.

The American Indians of the plains, such as the Cheyenne, Crow, Arapaho, Sioux, etc., show a high-bridged and often aquiline nose.

Malar Bone

Also called the zygomatic bones, bones of the cheek, they show a curving as they arch to the sides of the skull in both Caucasian and Negro skulls. In many Mongoloid skulls (not all) these bones are flatter and the arch to the sides of the skull is more at a right angle. This feature is particularly striking in the skulls of Plains Indians of the United States and Canada. The face on the living is broad. It is commonly referred to as "high cheek bones" and the "moon face" of many Chinese. This angling makes for a forward thrust of the malar bone, causing the inferior orbital border to be anterior to the superior, which is the reverse in Caucasians and Negroes.

The upper facial index values are quite revealing; this index derives from the following formula:

$$\frac{\text{upper facial height} \times 100}{\text{bizygomatic width}}$$

Upper facial height is measured from nasion (nasal root) to prosthion (point on the maxilla between the central incisor teeth). Bizygomatic width is the width across the cheek bones.

Hypereurene (very broad or low) .... 45% and lower
Euryene (broad) .... 45% to 49.9%
Mesene (medium) .... 50% to 54.9%
Leptene (narrow or high) .... 55% to 59.9%
Hyperleptene (very narrow) .... 60% and above.

The extremes of facial flatness are found among Eskimos and some tribes of Siberia, such as the Tungus. This facial flatness is enhanced in the living by fat pads over the cheeks, but the basic structure is present in the architecture of the facial skeleton.

Bony Brow Ridges

The development of bony ridges over the orbital rims was a well-developed trait in man of the ancient times, from some 50,-000 years ago and back. These ridges served a twofold purpose at the very least: (1) to protect the highly vulnerable and delicately structured eyes, and (2) as shunt for the lines of stress radiating up the face whenever the jaws were closed. In modern man, this feature shows its greatest development in the skulls of the Australian aborigines, both sexes. Next in size development are Europeans and their descendants, males only. It is rarely seen, if at all, in Negroes and Mongoloids of both sexes, with the exceptions of the Plains Indian males, where it is as marked as in European males.

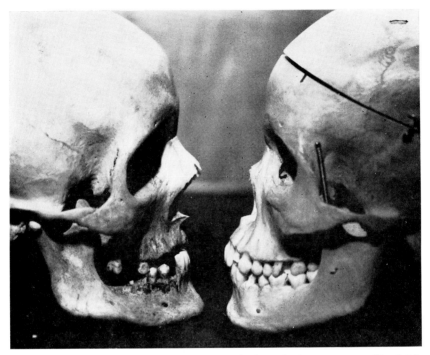

Figure 24. Distinct alveolar prognathism (right). Orthoganous profile (left). From Charles G. Wilber, *Forensic Biology for the Law Enforcement Officer,* 1974. Courtesy of Charles C Thomas, Publisher, Springfield, Illinois.

Prognathism

The Negro skull generally shows a marked alveolar prognathism, a forward jut of the mouth region beyond a line dropped from the brow or frontal bone. This trait is rare in Caucasians and somewhat more frequent in Mongoloids (Fig. 24).

Inca Bone

This is the name given to the back portion of the rear bone of the skull, the occipital, when it is divided in two large sections.

Its frequency is, oddly enough, greatest in the natives of the Melanesian Islands of New Britain and New Ireland in the Western Pacific, who are not Mongoloids. The frequency of the Inca bone in Europeans is 1.0 percent; Australian aborigines, 0.8 percent; African Negroes, 2.0 percent; Preconquest and Modern Peruvian Indians, 5.2 percent; Indians of Mexico, 5.6 percent; and Indians of the United States, up to 6.7 percent.

Os Japonicum

The so-called Japanese bone is the result of an extra suture that divides the malar or cheek bone into two or more sections. Again, we have the oddity of the highest frequency for this trait not in the Japanese but in the Ainu, who are Japanese Nationals but not of the Mongoloid race. It is next highest in Japanese, perhaps by the force of gene flow.

The following frequencies are taken from DeVilliers (1968):

Caucasoids .... up to 0.5%
South African Negroids 0.4%
American Indians .... up to 0.2%
Japanese .... up to 21.1%
Ainu .... up to 48.8%

Doctor Alice Brues, physical anthropologist now at the University of Colorado, Boulder, solved a most fascinating case of a skull in a paper sack in the attic of an Oklahoma City house. I have spelled out the details of the neat puzzler in another publication (Charney, 1974).

The Long Bones

The long bones of Caucasians are generally more massive, the muscular markings more prominent, and the joints larger.

The lengths of the bones in the leg and the arm show racial differences, though this phenomenon is variable with some overlap.

In Negroes, the lower sections, tibia in the leg and radius in the arm, are relatively longer with respect to their upper bones, the femur and humerus. This relationship is generally lowest in Mongoloids.

Stature Reconstruction

One does not always have the complete cadaver or skeleton in one piece for ease of determining stature. In fact, I have never had a case in which I was not forced to turn to the various regression formulas for the estimation of the stature from the lengths of the individual bones. These formulas have been derived by many workers; the best known and most widely used in the United States are those of Trotter and Gleser (1952, 1958). With the length of one or more long bones determined by measurement, one consults the regression formula table (Table VII) after analysis of the bones for sex and race. Genoves (1967) has prepared similar formulations for Mesoamerican Indians (Table VIII), and I have used them in analyses of American Indian skeletal remains with remarkable accuracy (Charney, 1974, pp. 319-324).

There are other such regression formulas for Germans, Finns, French, Irish, Italian, Portugese, Chinese, and East Indians (Krogman, 1962). Singh and Bhasin (1968) list tables for Maharashin males from India.

It is possible to arrive at a good approximation of stature even

TABLE VII

STATURE RECONSTRUCTION FROM LONG BONES*

MALES		
Caucasian	*Negro*	*Mongoloid*
1.31 (fem + fib) + 63.05	1.20 (fem + fib) + 67.7	1.22 (fem + fib) + 70.24
1.26 (fem + tib) + 67.09	1.15 (fem + tib) + 71.75	1.22 (fem + tib) + 70.37
2.60 fibula + 75.5	2.34 fibula + 80.07	2.40 fibula + 80.56
2.32 femur + 65.53	2.10 femur + 72.22	2.15 femur + 72.57
2.42 tibia + 81.93	2.19 tibia + 85.36	2.39 tibia + 81.45
1.82 (hum + rad) + 67.97	1.66 (hum + rad) + 73.08	1.67 (hum + rad) + 74.83
1.78 (hum + ulna) + 66.98	1.65 (hum + ulna) + 70.67	1.68 (hum + ulna) + 71.18
2.89 humerus + 78.10	2.88 humerus + 75.48	2.68 humerus + 83.19
3.79 radius + 79.43	3.32 radius + 85.43	3.54 radius + 82.00
3.76 ulna + 75.55	3.20 ulna + 82.77	3.48 ulna + 77.45

FEMALES	
Caucasian	*Negro*
0.68 hum + 1.17 fem + 1.15 tib + 50.12	0.44 hum + 0.20 rad + 1.46 fem + 0.86 tib + 56.33
1.39 (fem + tib) + 53.52	1.53 fem + 0.96 tib + 58.54
2.93 fibula + 59.61	2.49 fibula + 70.90
2.90 tibia + 61.53	2.45 tibia + 72.65
1.35 humerus + 1.95 tibia + 52.77	1.08 humerus + 1.79 tibia + 62.80
2.47 femur + 54.10	2.28 femur + 59.76
4.74 radius + 54.93	2.75 radius + 94.51
4.27 ulna + 57.76	3.31 ulna + 75.38
3.36 humerus + 57.97	3.08 humerus + 64.67

* From Trotter and Gleser (1952, 1958) .

TABLE VIII

STATURE RECONSTRUCTION FROM LONG BONES*

Males	
Femur	stature = 2.26 femur + 66.379 ± 3.417 (in cm)
Tibia	stature = 1.96 tibia + 93.752 ± 2.812
Females	
Femur	stature = 2.59 femur + 49.742 ± 3.816
Tibia	stature = 2.72 tibia + 63.781 ± 3.513

* From Genoves (1967). These formulas can be applied with great accuracy to American Indians of the Greater Southwest.

when all you have to work with is a fragment of a long bone. For a discussion of this with formulations, see Charney (1974, pp. 313-314).

Age at Time of Death

"Professor, how old would you say this person was when 'it' died?" A most reasonable request on the part of the constabulary, but it is one that can only be answered in a general way, with a plus-or-minus five years' range in adults and less in children.

Tooth eruption sequence is commonly used in the aging of children and adolescents (*see* Chap. 7).

In growth of all mammals, bones grow by replacement of cartilage at the ends by the bone cells. The ends of long bone have separate centers of ossification and thus are separated during growth from the shaft. The attainment of full growth means the ends and shaft are now all bone and the softer cartilage is gone.

There is a wealth of data on the growth rate of long bones in various populations, and these data show a great variability in the ages at which such growth is completed.

Figure 25 gives the kind of information you should look for when presented with a long bone that shows open ends or, if closed very recently, shows the line of closure. The dark, solid boxes indicate the age range of completion of bone growth for most people, termed the *Central Tendency*. These data are taken from Krogman (1962). The open, longer rectangles give the extreme ranges at which cessation of bone growth can occur.

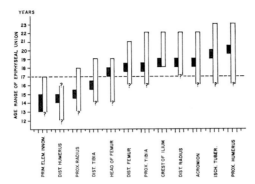

Figure 25. Age ranges in which various bones show closure or epiphyseal union.

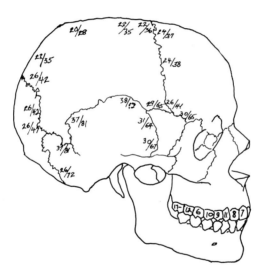

Figure 26. Suture closure of the skull. Upper figures denote onset of closure, lower figures give age of obliteration. Asterisk indicates that the suture never closes. The figures on the upper teeth denote the usual age in years of permanent teeth eruption. Caution is advised in the use of these figures owing to the great variability involved. From Charles G. Wilber, *Forensic Biology for the Law Enforcement Officer,* 1974. Courtesy of Charles C Thomas, Publisher, Springfield, Illinois.

These data come from McKern and Stewart (1957). You may consult various standard textbooks of anatomy, such as Cunningham and Gray, for information on growth rates of other bones.

The appearance of the face of the pubic symphysis changes through life, and detailed data on this phenomenon exist for both American males and females. This is not a technique to be attempted by the beginner or amateur. In this case, it is best to consult with a physical anthropologist skilled in osteology.

On the skull, the sutures at the meeting lines of the various bones show changes with advancing years. The sutures close and obliterate, but unfortunately, too many skulls do not follow any sequential order and, in fact, never close. Because of this, many competent workers in this field will not use suture closure rates of the skull as an aid in aging. It has been my practice in disaster identification to use any and all information, including skull suture closure where such closure and obliteration occur.

Figure 26 shows the years of suture closure onset and obliteration from different parts of the skull. The figures along the top of the skull refer to the sagittal suture, not visible in this drawing.

Bone Pathology and Injury

Quite apart from injury to bone as the result of violence, mayhem, and accident, there are several diseases that leave their trademark on bone. Arthritis is probably the first to come to mind, both rheumatoid and osteoarthritic forms. Tuberculosis, yaws, syphilis, and osteomyelitis are other diseases that mark bone. Also, there are such diet deficiency syndromes as rickets and osteomalacia, bone tumors and deformities due to infantile paralysis, congenital hip dysplasia, and endocrine disturbances such as hyper- and hypopituitary function, which cause acromegaly and dwarfism.

The above are but a few of the abnormal states that affect bone. All such detail can be most important in an identity case. The police officer should not hesitate to avail himself of the assistance of experts in this field.

The decay of tooth and its treatment affords the investigator a useful tool for individualizing an unknown skeleton or body. This subject is more fully treated in the chapter on forensic dentistry.

In the case of the Shoshone woman discussed in Charney (1972), the nasal bones showed a series of fracture lines. The husband of the woman had been a Golden Gloves boxer and was known to have beaten his wife when intoxicated. However, the nasal bones alone were broken, not other facial bones, as would be expected if the above story were the basis for the lopsided nose. Then it was learned that the woman had been in a car mishap, and at the sudden halt of forward movement of the car, she kept going, her nose making sudden and violent contact with the edge of the dashboard. Now the nature of the nasal bone fractures and left deviation made sense.

Bones Mistaken for Human

Hardly a week goes by without some specimen being brought to me for analysis by students, the public, or the constabulary. In most cases, these are not human and the bearer is so aware, but not always. In most cases of mistaken identity, it is merely unfamiliarity with basic skeletal morphology. In the case of the foot and hand of a bear, the resemblance to the human structure is so close as to fool all but the expert. To be sure, no one would be so fooled if the skin and claws were present. However, the hunter skins the animal, and the claws go with the skin. Then the hands and feet are generally sawn and left behind for someone else to find. With whitened face and horror-filled eyes, he reports to the local sheriff that a fiendish mutilating killer has left a clue.

Disaster Identification

In the summer of 1976, I was involved, as deputy coroner, in the identification of the victims of the Big Thompson Canyon flood disaster of Larimer County, Colorado. Doctor Patrick Allen and I were given the responsibility of the operation of the temporary morgue and the task of individual identification of the victims.

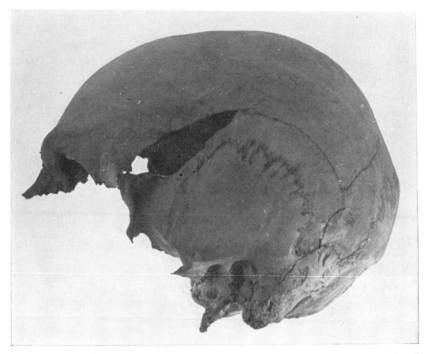

Figure 27. Skull of victim #129 from the Big Thompson Canyon flood disaster.

The herculean efforts of the deputy sheriffs, struggling in the rugged mountainous terrain and frightful wreckage, made for swift recovery of the bodies. To date, one hundred and thirty-nine bodies have been recovered and identified. Fifty percent of the bodies were brought out in the first two days, 60 percent by the first week, another 14 percent by the second week, and 14 percent again by the third week. This swift action enabled us to study bodies with little deterioration of tissue. Later, the action of the agents of destruction meant that data relating to age, sex, and stature would have to come from a study of the bones. Most of the bodies were incomplete, limbs and portions of the skulls missing.

The individual identification of body #129 should be of interest. The postcranial remains were a mangled mess of badly necrotic tissue and broken bones. The skull was missing the facial and basal portions. Sex and stature estimates were obtained from the appropriate bones, as outlined earlier in this chapter. Age was put at over seventy years. We had few males listed as missing in this age bracket. One missing person folder contained some ten x-ray plates made nine years previously. Figures 27, 28, 29, and 30 tell the story. You can see that the outline of the skull in lateral view matches that of the x-ray of Mr. C.S.; Figure 29 shows the x-ray superimposed on the skull. The frontal views show the outline of the frontal sinuses. No two people would have the same configuration. The match of the sinuses of body #129 and that of Mr. C.S. is perfect.

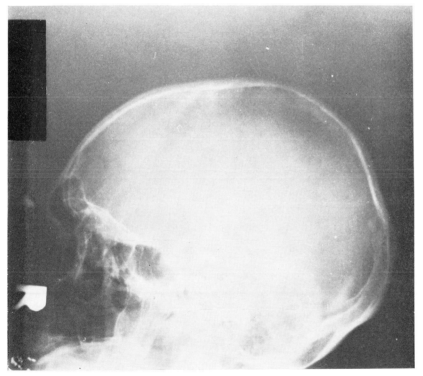

Figure 28. X-ray of the skull of one of the missing persons in the Big Thompson Canyon flood. The photo had been taken nine years prior to the flood.

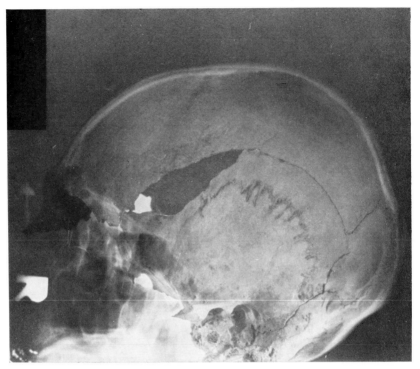

Figure 29. X-ray in Figure 28 superimposed on the skull in Figure 27.

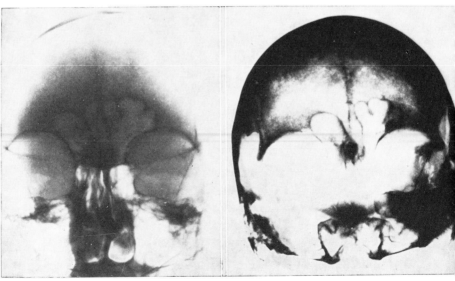

Figure 30. View of the frontal sinuses of body #129 and the missing person.

Conclusion

The physical anthropologist trained in skeletal morphology is an expert any law enforcement agency can call on when needed. Our speciality does not contain numerous individuals; as mentioned, there are only twenty-eight members of the Physical Anthropology section of the American Academy of Forensic Sciences, but we are spread across the nation and easily contacted. We will not only address ourselves to the specific case at hand but will be glad to explain as we work to the interested law enforcement officer. At Colorado State University, I have taught numerous workshops and the like to the constabulary. In actual disaster identification cases submitted by various law enforcement agencies in Texas, New Jersey, Idaho, and Colorado since 1938, I have never asked for (nor have I received) a fee for services rendered. I have always considered this work a public service.

CHAPTER 7

Forensic Odontology

MICHAEL CHARNEY

It was back in 1939. A call came into the Scientific Crime Detection Laboratory of Headquarters, Department of Public Safety, State of Texas, from the police at Waxahachie. They wanted someone from the bureau to aid in a case of breaking, entry, and robbery of a grocery. A block of cheese turned up with a set of teeth marks. Someone evidently did not care for the flavor and backed his mouth out the way it went into the cheese.

It was a most unusual bite, quite out of the ordinary. A check of the dental records in the town, and a local lad was quickly arrested. Many years later, on June 4, 1972, a syndicated Sunday news supplement, *Parade,* carried a short article telling exactly the same story, but in a town in West Germany. The article was headed "New Clue" and was full of wonderment and praise for the cleverness of the German police.

[Postscript: I wrote to the editor of *Parade,* telling him of the Texas incident of thirty-three years back in a town unpronounceable to non-Texans. I never received a reply!]

THE ABOVE CASE illustrates one of the subfields within the fascinating field of forensic odontology, or the application of dental science to legal problems. Three broad areas of study are encompassed within forensic odontology. In addition to the investigation of bite marks, on people as well as cheese, the field also includes the examination of dental remains as an aid in individual identification. Finally, the science also includes the examination and interpretation of injuries to the teeth and other oral tissues. For example, intentional beatings of children sometimes may be diagnosed on the nature and extent of injuries to the mouth and teeth.

In investigation of a criminal nature, or of mass disasters and the like, teeth and jaws are a source of detailed, individualized information, where restorations have been made. Dental records can pinpoint the exact locations of all fillings and the nature of the material used in the filling. The dental journals regularly carry photographs of dental x-rays that are seeking recognition by some home-town dentist. Navy dentists use dental records to aid in the identification of sailors who had fallen into the sea and whose bodies were not recovered for several weeks.

Even severely burnt human remains have been identified by the remaining teeth and bridgework. Johanson and Saldeen (1969) describe three cases in Sweden that truly make fact more fascinating than fiction.

Teeth in Age Determination

The eruption of deciduous teeth is a subject of concern to many parents. Much emphasis is placed upon the timetables set forth in the child-care literature. If a child's tooth erupts two months before the specified date, the parents are likely to be filled with pride; a delay of two months in the eruption of the same tooth can cause needless worry or even embarrassment.

In reality, there is no such thing as a fixed schedule for deciduous tooth eruption, but people in general are only aware of what is called the central tendency, the "average" date, for the appearance of the deciduous or baby teeth. There is quite a range of normal eruption time for all teeth, with minor variation between boys and girls. The forensic scientist who does not take these ranges into consideration is no forensic scientist.

Table IX gives the central tendency and ranges for the eruption of both sets, deciduous and permanent, in American Caucasians.

The tooth eruption sequence does not show significant differences in the several races to be of sufficient value to warrant listing. Work on Japanese suggests that the upper canines emerge earlier than in Caucasians on the average.

Hurme (1957) states that largely unverified data on African blacks suggests an eruptive process from one-half to one and one-half years earlier than in Europeans and European-derived populations.

Bang and Ramm (1970) have published on an age-determination technique based on the degree of root dentine transparency. Because of the importance of assessing the age of a body, a small discussion of the technique of Bang and Ramm is warranted.

TABLE IX

TOOTH ERUPTION SEQUENCE

Maxillary Teeth

	Central Tendency	Range Male	Female
Deciduous			
Medial incisors	9-12 mos.	4-15 mos.	4-15 mos.
Lateral incisors	12-14	5-19	6-20
First molars	15-16	9-22	9-22
Canines	20-24	9-27	11-28
Second molars	30-32	8-35	6-37
Permanent			
First molars	6- 7 yrs.	4.75-8.75 yrs.	4.25- 8.50 yrs.
Medial incisors	7- 8	4.75-9.25	5.25- 8.75
Lateral incisors	8- 9	6.25-11.0	
Premolar #1	9-12	7.50-13.75	7.25-13.25
Premolar #2	10-12	8.25-14.0	7.75-14.0
Canines	11-12	8.25-13.75	8.0 -13.25
Second molars	12-13	9.25-15.0	9.5 -15.0

Mandibular Teeth

	Central Tendency	Range Male	Female
Deciduous			
Medial incisors	6- 8 mos.	2-15 mos.	2-14 mos.
Lateral incisors	14-15	5-20	5-20
First molars	15-16	10-22	7-21
Canines	20-24	11-27	10-26
Second molars	30-32	15-32	15-34
Permanent			
First molars	6- 8 yrs.	4.25- 8.5 yrs.	4.25- 8.75 yrs.
Medial incisors	7- 8	4.75- 8.25	4.50- 8.0
Lateral incisors	8- 9	5.50- 9.25	5.00- 8.75
Premolar #1	9-12	7.50-13.5	6.75-13.5
Premolar #2	10-12	8.25-14.0	7.75-14.5
Canines	11-12	7.75-13.25	7.00-12.5
Second molars	12-13	9.25-14.5	8.75-14.76
Third molars	18 and one, if at all		

The root dentin appears to become transparent during the third decade of life. The process begins at the tip of the root and advances towards the crown with age. Bang and Ramm measured the length of root transparency on intact roots and/or on longitudinal sections of roots.

Over 1,000 teeth were measured. The authors observed a significant increase in root transparency with age. The length of the transparency could not be determined in only 5.3 percent of the intact roots and in 1.6 percent of the longitudinal root sections. In all, teeth from 265 subjects covering ages from approximately 20 to 80 years formed the study sample. The method is simple enough so that it could easily be applied by others without previous extensive training or expensive equipment.

There was some tendency to underestimate age in elderly people. The authors discussed the application of the method in three actual cases. I cite one of these below.

The decomposed body of a male was found hanging in a tree. Five teeth were measured for age, giving estimates of 56.8, 57.2, 57.3, 59.4, and 60.5 years, for an estimated age of 58.2 years. This specimen was later identified; the man had been 56.0 years at the time of death.

Racing

In general, marked racial differences in teeth, save for upper incisor shoveling, are not evident from the studies to date. Tratman (1950) has a long and fascinating paper on a comparison of the teeth of Mongoloid and Caucasian peoples. He covers the subject tooth by tooth, deciduous and permanent, but his conclusions are not of a nature to be useful to the forensic scientist concerned with identification, excepting, to be sure, that of the shovel-shaped upper incisors.

Klatsky (1956) reports on the incidence of such dental traits as supernumerary teeth, congenitally missing teeth, peg teeth, impacted teeth, Carabelli cusps, protostylids, and the like for twenty-five human breeding groups and concludes that the frequencies of these anomalies are too uniform to be of any use in raciation.

The one characteristic that does stand out in determining race affiliation is the above-mentioned shoveling of the upper incisors, a term introduced into the literature by Hrdlicka, late curator of physical anthropology at the Smithsonian. Shoveling refers to a buildup of extra enamel on the lateral margins of the incisors. It is a feature of our early ancestors, serving to extend the life of the upper incisors. Figure 31 shows marked shoveling of these teeth. Also note the crowding of the front teeth, but the abun-

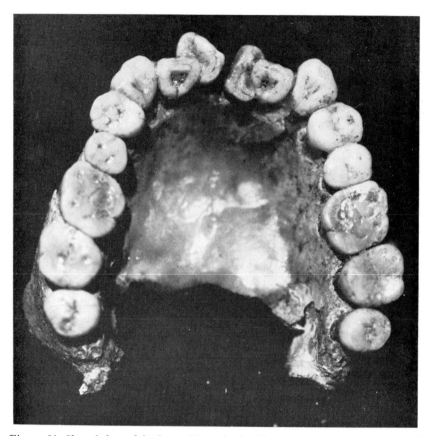

Figure 31. Shovel-shaped incisors: Note the build-up of enamel on the lateral margins of the incisors and even the canines of the upper palate. Note too, the crowding of the incisors. From Charles G. Wilber, *Forensic Biology for the Law Enforcement Officer,* 1974. Courtesy of Charles C Thomas, Publisher, Springfield, Illinois.

dance of room for the three molars. Such crowding of the incisors is the more common occurrence.

Dahlberg (1951) gives detailed frequency on the incidence of shoveling, separately for the medial and lateral incisors, and in several breeding populations. Carbonell (1963) arrives at much the same data and brings up a point about the evaluation of the degree of shoveling. A quantification is generally given in all reports, such as marked, moderate, slight, and trace. For categories such as "slight" and "trace," a degree of subjectivity is unavoidable, and this is unfortunate. Carbonell asks for some standardization of methodology in the estimation of the degree of shoveling.

In general, the frequency for shoveled incisors is very high in Mongoloid peoples, ranging from 75 to 100 percent for most American Indian groups. In Caucasians, it is about 9 percent and in Negroes about 11 percent.

Other than the shoveled upper incisors, what else can be said about dental variations of racial significance? Remember that there is no such thing as an exclusive racial marker, that rather we have varying frequencies of a trait, higher in some groups and low in others.

In general, big people have large teeth and small people have small teeth. Australian aborigines, American Indians, Eskimos, and Melanesians and Polynesians have large teeth with long, wide crowns. Bushmen, Lapps, and Siberians (not the European Russians of the famous salt mines) are small people and are small toothed. Europeans and European-derived peoples vary a great deal. American blacks on the average have large crown measurements.

Relative dimensions are also helpful in a general way in assigning race. Lasker (1950) gives several sources for the following: The second molar in Australian aborigines tends to be the longest, whereas in most people the size order decreases from the first to the third molars. Eskimos have large molars by comparison with average-sized premolars and anterior teeth. In Caucasians, the lateral upper incisor tends to be of smaller size than the medials. In Mongoloids, this size difference between the upper incisors tends not to be so great. In the Australian aborigine, the roots go deep. Bushmen have deep roots in contrast to low crowns; shallow roots and high crowns are found in the Lapps, and the Japanese have shallow roots both absolutely and relatively.

Lasker also covers much of Tratmen's data and that of others in an analysis of racial variations, such as they are, in each tooth.

He points up the isolated nature of these studies, the gaps in coverage, the dearth of comparative studies, and that these isolated studies are of little interest to the forensic scientist because much of the data employed methods that do not permit direct comparisons.

Lasker concludes that in general, Europeans and their descendants show the highest frequencies of chisel-shaped incisors, Carabelli cusps, and bent and splayed roots of the molars. Mongoloids, in addition to the shovel-shaped upper incisors, show the highest frequencies of enamel extensions onto the roots, enamel pearls, taurodont molars, and fused roots. Negro teeth have still to be studied in any great detail. If all this sounds at odds with Klatsky's remarks, it is. As a forensic anthropologist, I use every scrap of information that will build up the evidence towards an identification.

In addition to having influences on the morphology of teeth, racial characteristics also may be reflected in the way dentists make fillings and other dental restorations. Pedersen and Keiser-Nielsen (1961) found that fillings and restorations often differed from country to country and therefore might be useful for identification purposes. They at least might furnish some information about the country of origin of the dentist, although there doesn't appear to have been any detailed work in the technique and material utilized by dentists in different countries.

Camps (1953) described a case in which the dental restoration played an important role in determining the race of a victim. An artificial crown was of a type known as a "shell crown" and made of a silver palladium alloy. This type of crown and alloy is not common in England but is utilized in central Europe. It was thought reasonable to deduce that this one was probably of central European origin. In conjunction with other evidence, the police suspected that the remains were those of an Austrian girl.

Sexing by Teeth

There is not too much to go on when it comes to determining the sex by teeth alone. Attempts to sex a specimen by the teeth without prior knowledge of the age can be terribly misleading.

The permanent canines erupt much earlier in females than in

males—by as much as eleven months. Hurme (1957) says that as a general rule, in children where the maxillary canine erupts close to or prior to the maxillary second premolar, it is safe to assume you are dealing with a female rather than a male. The Japanese show this same phenomenon.

At the twenty-eighth annual meeting of the American Academy of Forensic Sciences, held in Washington, D.C. the week of February 16, 1976, a paper read at the physical anthropology section gave out that a close correlation in the estimation of age between bone growth and tooth development generally meant a female, whereas a greater gap between the two estimates of age meant you were dealing with a male child. It was claimed that an accuracy of 75 percent could be obtained by this technique. It certainly bears further study, for at present one does not attempt a sexing of a preadolescent with any confidence.

A Word on the Genetics of Teeth

Some understanding of the evolution of human jaws and teeth might help make the modern scene clearer. Our hominid ancestors, the Australopithecines, the Pithecanthropines (more properly known as Homo erectus), and the Neanderthals (called Homo sapiens neanderthalensis), all had terrifically large jaws and teeth compared to man of today, though the teeth were relatively small in comparison to the bony jaw. Both the jaws and teeth were reducing throughout the millions of years of human evolution. As Goose (1963; 143) puts it, "one might expect to find a close correlation between jaws and teeth since they are related functionally and presumably have some common genetic control." However, the "common genetic control" either slipped a bit or was at best a tenuous one, for in recent man the jaws have reduced faster and further than the teeth, with a resulting disharmony that is still occurring in so-called civilized groups. Hooton (1946) believes that this trend accelerated under the impact of urban living and cereal diets.

Goose says that a comparison of British skulls of the Roman occupation era shows a harmony between jaws and teeth with no undue crowding. In modern jaws, the crowding of teeth is more often the rule.

Dental Identification in Mass Disaster

Whatever its causes, the decay of teeth calls for attempts to prolong their use-life by repair. It is not usual to find any two people with such dental repair to be exactly alike. Add to this the selective loss of teeth, and one's mouth begins to take on the individualization of fingerprints. For purposes of identification, the teeth are superior to fingerprints because of their hardness. What we know of the fossil record of apes and monkeys of tens of millions of years back is due to persistence of teeth and jaws when all other bones have long since deteriorated.

And so, in mass disaster, or even in single cases, as mentioned earlier, where any of the victims have some dental restoration, fillings, and the like, individual positive identification is possible. However, it is not possible to depend solely on the dental picture, for the older populations are more prone to be toothless and the very young cavity free or, at best, total strangers to the dentist chair.

Other factors may also enter to thwart an identification by dental means. In a most recent case, I sent to a dental journal complete x-rays and photographs of extensive dental repair—all upper and lower molars, eight in all, had occlusal fillings, the right upper canine more than two-thirds filled with porcelain held in place by two brass pins or studs, and an upper left lateral incisor porcelain faced with a gold crown. All this in a woman of only twenty-six years. No dentist called us to say he recognized the picture. Positive identification was made by a facial reconstruction in clay, recognized by the mother in a telecast. Where was the dentist? He went on holiday the very month the x-rays and photographs were listed in the dental journal. To be sure, he later corroborated the identification.

In air crashes, where death is accompanied by severe destruction of tissue due to burning, dental examinations have played a major role in identifying the victims. Haines (1972) tells that fifty of the seventy-eight dead in a plane crash in Yugoslavia in 1971 were identified by dental restorations, orthodontal work, specially constructed dentures, and, surprisingly enough, names on denture plates. Thus, on the order of 64 percent of all the victims were so identified. However, Haines includes seven victims where just the age was deduced from the teeth. Even so, with these seven left out, a 53.8 percent record is remarkable.

In 1969, the Connecticut State Dental Association formed a volunteer dental disaster squad. Luntz and Luntz (1972) describe the work of this unit in helping to identify the victims of an air crash in New Haven in June, 1971, where twenty-eight of the thirty-one passengers perished. Again, as in the Yugoslavia crash, there was severe burning of the bodies.

The literature contains many papers on the contributions of dental science to problems of identification.

The Big Thompson Canyon flood of July 31, 1976, that has yielded 139 dead to date, profited greatly by the sterling work of Lieutenant Colonel William Morlang, USAF, and Staff Sergeant Wright, USAF, both members of the forensic dental unit that responds to service air crashes. Morlang worked closely with Doctor Allen and myself in a team approach to identification. A total description of the corpse was made, then we searched for some trait or aspect that would individualize the corpse. Dental examination was responsible for 25 percent of the identifications. Few of the children and adolescents had dental records, and the elderly were edentulous—completely toothless.

The case that was especially intriguing, body #139, the last victim to be found so far, was represented only by facial bones. Some adhering strands of hair gave one clue; the erupting first permanent molar and crown formation of the second permanent molar provided a second clue—one that gave an indication of age (Fig. 32).

Now we were in luck. That child had been to the dentist, and an x-ray film of the anterior teeth was in the victim's chart. They showed the crowns of the permanent central incisors in their sockets, teeth that would not erupt for a few years. I asked Doctor Harden, of Loveland, one of our team of local dentists working with Morlang, to x-ray the fragment of the skull. A comparison of the two x-rays (Fig. 33) left no doubt as to the identity of body #139.

In summation, the following statements can be made:

1. Do not be misled by using average eruption time for the in-

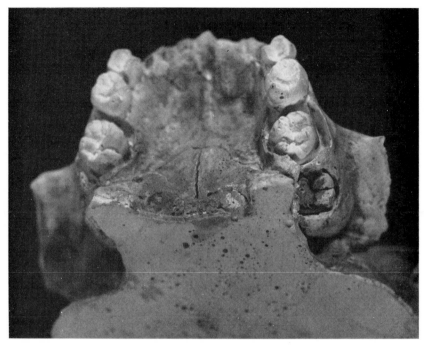

Figure 32. Teeth of victim #139 of the Big Thompson Canyon flood disaster. Note the erupting first permanent molar and the crown formation of the second permanent molar. These features indicate the teeth are from a child. Photograph by Mark J. Riedo.

dividual teeth. Be aware of the upper and lower limits of time. Use all the teeth you have, not just one or two.

2. It is highly dangerous to age by teeth where the sex is not known. Where you are working with preadolescents, use estimates of long bone age and dental age as an aid in sexing, if you must.

3. Remember that eruption of teeth need not follow the usual order and frequently does not.

4. Forget the third molar (the "Wisdom" tooth). You will be no wiser in your estimate of age from this notoriously variable tooth.

5. Racial differences in tooth morphology rely mostly in diagnosing a Mongoloid by the shovel-shaped upper incisors.

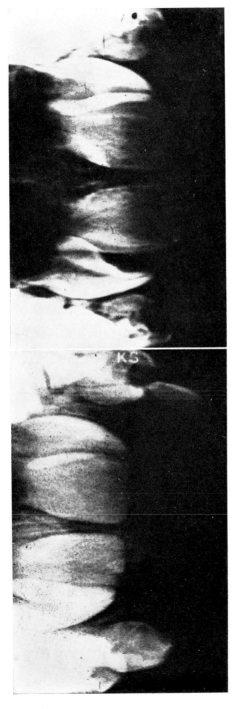

Figure 33. Comparison of x-rays of the anterior teeth of victim #139 and those of a child missing in the Big Thompson Canyon flood. Note that the crowns of the permanent central incisors are in their sockets in both cases. Photograph by Mark J. Riedo and Cliff Nicholson.

Differences in eruption sequences have not been too well investigated. Only African blacks are thought to be precocious on this point.

Certification in Forensic Odontology

The increasing application of odontology to the forensic sciences is reflected in the recent initiation of a program of certification in forensic odontology by the American Board of Forensic Odontology. As stated by the Board, the requisite background for certification includes the following:

1. good moral character and high ethical and professional standing
2. acceptable education
3. acceptable recent professional experience in forensic odontology

Details of the standards are provided in the Board's statement on "Qualifications and Requirements for Certification in Forensic Odontology." These qualifications and requirements may be looked upon as a possible model for other specialties in forensic science. When one realizes what may be at stake in the application of science to legal problems, it is imperative that quality and competence be beyond reproach.

CHAPTER 8

Blood and Other Body Fluids*

S INCE THE FIRST application of blood grouping in court cases in the 1920s, forensic serology has assumed an ever-increasing role in the resolution of medicolegal problems. Today, more and more forensic testing laboratories and laboratories of crime detection are including sections devoted to serology and immunohematology. Techniques are applied to problems in the identification of individuals, the establishment of familiar relationships, paternity testing, and the identification of bloodstains, blood crusts, bone, hair, saliva, semen, and fingernails. It is felt that the modern law enforcement officer should have a basic appreciation and understanding of the importance of forensic serology to the various problems of individual identity. It is the goal of this chapter to present a brief review of forensic serology, with an emphasis on its application to the identification of bloodstains and other body secretions. It is not the intention of this chapter to provide the reader with the methodologies and techniques that are utilized in forensic serology. It might be too easy to infer from a mere presentation of such "technical recipes" that proficiency in the utilization of the techniques is readily acquired.

Who is qualified to serve as an "expert" in the application of forensic serology? There is at present no agreement as to the requirements. Moreover, there is no agency responsible for the certification of qualifications such as are found in a number of clinical sciences, including clinical pathology and blood banking.

Craycroft et al. (1971) have suggested the following criteria for qualifications of forensic scientists:

1. Medical technologist or equivalent
2. Reference laboratory experience—two years
3. Forensic laboratory experience—one to two years

---

* Modified from Charles G. Wilber, *Forensic Biology for the Law Enforcement Officer*, 1974. Courtesy of Charles C Thomas, Publisher, Springfield, Illinois.

4. Continuing education to include
   A. Formal training—genetics, cytogenetics, biochemistry, and immunohematology, leading to advanced degrees
   B. Liaison with other forensic testing laboratories
   C. Attendance at forensic conferences
   D. Review of the literature in forensic sciences

Similar types of guidelines have been suggested by a committee of forensic medical experts in East Germany (Prokop and Uhlenbruck, 1969) who proposed that a practitioner have the following minimum standards of qualifications:

1. At least five years of training and practice in the field of blood group serology under the supervision of an expert who himself is government licensed.
2. Complete knowledge of Wiener's nomenclature especially and of the genetic problems of all systems.
3. Evidence that he has carried out scientific investigations on his own.
4. The passing of an examination set by a government committee.

For designation as a practitioner in charge, both ten years experience in the field of blood group serology and a knowledge of anthropology are required in addition.

The above authors have stressed that such qualifications should be regarded as the very minimum requirements. It is easy to appreciate the significance of rigid requirements when one realizes the consequences of incorrect conclusions stemming from incorrectly performed tests. Such errors may lead readily to miscarriages of justice. It is therefore essential that a forensic scientist be able to guarantee complete accuracy and reliability in his technical procedures. It is not sufficient for a laboratory to merely know how certain methods are employed. Forensic science experts know that continued practice and experience in the utilization of a technique or test are essential if the proper level of proficiency is to be maintained. By analogy, a sharpshooter cannot rest on his laurels but must constantly practice to maintain his proficiency at shooting. Laboratory proficiency is no different. Most clinical laboratories in hospitals have the capability to carry out routine blood grouping tests that might be necessary for operations or transfusions. It is doubtful, however, if the same laboratories, without prior experience, could be expected to carry out successful forensic testing in specialized applications such as ABO typing of bone, for example.

The Biology of the ABO Blood Groups

The basic genetics of the ABO blood groups were covered in Chapter 1. The ABO system continues to have extensive medicolegal applications, and it has been widely used in problems of individual identification. ABO blood groups have been identified from a variety of sources, including fresh blood, bloodstains, semen, saliva, bone, and even inner ear fluid!

The differences between the red blood cells of one individual and those of another are due to differences in the chemical structures, called blood group antigens, on the cell surface. Numerous different red cell antigens have been reported. Since each of the different antigens is the result of a different inherited gene, any single individual is likely to represent a unique combination of antigens due to the extremely large number of combinations of genes that can be inherited. For the most part, the specific biological functions of the red cell antigens are not known.

Nomenclature of the ABO blood groups is based upon the antigen which is present on the erythrocytes or red cells. In general terms, an antigen may be any substance which has the power to elicit the formation of an antibody when injected into another organism that is not immunologically compatible. Antibodies usually are highly specific for the antigen against which they are produced. When serum from one person is mixed with red cells from another person who is not compatible, the red cells will form into clumps or clusters or are said to agglutinate. ABO blood group phenotypes are distinguished on the basis of this agglutination reaction.

Characteristic of the ABO blood groups is the reciprocal relation that exists between the antigens that are present on the red cells and the antibodies that occur in that same person's serum. (Refer to Table I, Chapter 2). The blood grouping chemicals or reagents that are used to determine a person's blood type or phenotype are sera that contain antibodies that are specific for different blood group antigens. Thus, anti-B serum contains antibodies that are specific and will agglutinate only red cells which have antigen B.

Other Blood Variations

The ABO system is only one of a number of blood group systems. Other blood group systems include the Rhesus (Rh), MN, Lewis, Kell, Lutheran, Kidd, I, P, Vel, Diego, Xg, Bu, Yt, and Duffy.

In addition to the individual differences observed in the cellular antigens of the above blood groups, individual genetic differences are also known to occur in hemoglobin (Fig. 34), blood proteins, and blood enzymes. Aside from the ABO, Rh, and MN systems, the other variants have not been utilized extensively in forensic serology. The genetics of some of these variants and the clinical ease and reliability of their detection are as good as those of the ABO system, and there is no real reason why they should not achieve equal medicolegal applications. Forensic scientists outside of the United States have been faster than their American counterparts to utilize different systems. The monograph by Culliford (1971) has described a number of applications of techniques to typing of bloodstains. The utilization of several different systems increases the precision with which individuals may be identified.

Utilization of Blood Group Frequency Data

Frequencies of the different blood group phenotypes vary in different populations or groups of people (Table X). Anthropologists have thus made use of serological data to classify the minor and major racial groups of humans. In certain popula-

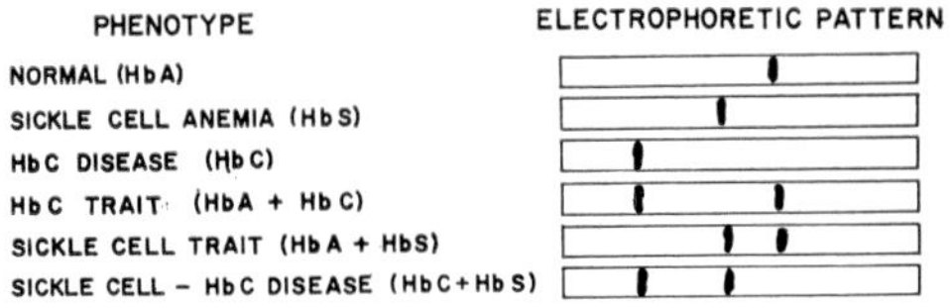

PHENOTYPE	ELECTROPHORETIC PATTERN
NORMAL (Hb A)	
SICKLE CELL ANEMIA (Hb S)	
Hb C DISEASE (Hb C)	
Hb C TRAIT (Hb A + Hb C)	
SICKLE CELL TRAIT (Hb A + Hb S)	
SICKLE CELL – Hb C DISEASE (Hb C + Hb S)	

Figure 34. Example of starch gel electrophoresis illustrating hemoglobin differences.

TABLE X

FREQUENCIES OF HUMAN BLOOD GROUPS*

Blood Group Phenotype	Caucasian %	Negro %
A	40.63	27.66
B	10.07	19.90
AB	3.70	3.33
O	45.58	49.09

* From Zmijewski and Fletcher (1972).

tions, specific blood types may be extremely rare or even lacking entirely.

Given a sample of blood such as a bloodstain, the problem lies in assessing the chance that a particular individual could have the same type of blood as found in the stain. For this purpose, one needs to calculate from population data the frequency of occurrence of the particular combinations of groups obtained.

Culliford (1971) has published the following data for blood group frequencies from British population data.

Blood Group	Frequency (%)
B	8.6
N	22.0
Ro	2.0
PGM 2	7.0
AK 2-1	7.0
ADA 2-1	11.0

These figures mean that 8.6 percent of the British population would belong to the blood group B (of the ABO system), 22.0 percent would belong to blood group N (of the MN system), etc. If the different systems are independent of each other, the frequency of an individual belonging to two or more specific groups is obtained by multiplying the separate frequencies. For example, the frequency of finding a person who was B and N would be 8.6% times 22.0% or 1.892%. The chance of finding a person with the six blood groups above would be approximately one in 5 million for the British population.

Now if the six blood groups were typed in a bloodstain, and if a "prime" suspect also belonged to the same six blood groups, the evidence, as in the example of disputed paternity discussed earlier, does not prove that the suspect left the bloodstain. It does indicate that it is "suspicious" that such a rare occurrence just happened to have been found in the suspect. In conjunction with other evidence, a court might decide that the suspect did or did not leave the bloodstain in question. Note again that as in the case of disputed paternity, if the blood type of the suspect does not match up identically with that of the bloodstain, it is possible to say that the suspect could not have left that particular bloodstain.

Unfortunately, as indicated earlier, most of the genetically controlled variants present in blood have not been utilized appreciably in forensic serology. Landsteiner predicted early in the development of serology that it should be possible to get a complete serologic profile of man. In other words, by typing of individuals for a number of blood variants, it should be possible to distinguish unique combinations for every individual that would be distinguishable from those same combinations of every other individual. In effect, a chemical fingerprint of blood could be produced for every person, and it would be as distinct as the classical physical fingerprints. It is not yet possible, or at least practicable, to do this, even when sufficient quantities of blood are available for testing. The forensic testing laboratory may be faced with the problem of working with a relatively small amount of material such as may be present in a bloodstain and must decide which blood tests should be selected on the basis of the circumstances of the particular case they are studying.

Recent Progress in the "Fingerprinting" of Blood

Although the research on blood groups and blood typing has yielded some spectacular results, the individualization or "fingerprinting" of human bloodstains has not yet been fully realized. The standard typing methods, even though some excellent methods requiring only minute quantities of blood have been developed, leave much to be desired when faced with the practical difficulties in the typing of limited amounts of blood present in a bloodstain.

Recently, Sweet and Elvins (1976) utilized a technique known as crossed electroimmunodiffusion to determine the individuality of bloodstains from different persons. The technique enables both qualitative and quantitative distinctions to be made of blood. Whitehead et al. (1970) had determined earlier that eluted bloodstain antigens are reactive and apparently distinguishable by crossed electroimmunodiffusion. Sweet and Elvins examined forty-eight-hour bloodstains from ten different individuals on ten different occasions. The crossed electroimmunodiffusion patterns revealed that there was at least one peak with a unique range in height which made it possible to achieve an individualization of the stains. In addition to the differences among individuals, statistically significant differences were observed among males and females, indicating that the technique may be useful in ascertaining the probability of a bloodstain having come from a male or a female.

Sweet and Elvins had utilized forty-eight-hour stains on the assumption that most crimes of violence ordinarily are discovered and reported within that interval. In addition, they examined some stains that were sixteen days old. Although some of the antigens were no longer resolved, it nevertheless was still possible to identify individuals. The overall results of this study indicate that the technique of crossed electroimmunodiffusion has a great potential for applications in forensic science.

ABO Secretor System

Of particular importance to the forensic scientist is the fact that the A and B antigens may also be present in a variety of tissues and other body fluids and secretions, including saliva, semen, and tears, in addition to being found on the red blood cells. Not all individuals (only about 80%) have the antigens present in the other body fluids. People who have antigens in these fluids are known as secretors, and their antigens exist in an alcohol-soluble form in the cells and a water-soluble form in the secretions. The remaining people have only the alcohol-soluble form in the cells.

The presence or absence of antigens in the secretions is genetically controlled, and the expression depends upon a single pair of genes that are inherited independently of genes of the ABO system. The so-called secretor gene (Se) is dominant over the nonsecretor gene (se). For example, in an individual with the genotype i^Ai^ASe Se, it would be possible to detect A antigens in the saliva, but A antigens would not be detectable in the saliva of an individual with the genotype i^Ai^Ase se.

The secretor-nonsecretor system increases the possibilities of individual identification for the forensic scientist through the utilization of these other types of fluids. For example, in rape cases, a seminal stain may be an important piece of evidence, and if the suspect genetically is a secretor, it may be possible to determine his ABO blood type from the seminal stain. It cannot be emphasized too strongly again, as in the cases discussed above, that a positive test does not by itself prove that a suspect did leave the stain but only that the evidence does not exclude him as a possibility.

Inner Ear Fluid

In attempting to do blood grouping of corpses, difficulties may arise if hemolysis has set in or if the corpse has been dismembered or has begun to decompose. In such cases, indirect methods of typing, including absorption and elution, which have been discussed earlier, have to be utilized. In many cases, these techniques have been unable to yield positive results.

Trela and Turowska (1975) reported very interesting results from a study of ABO group substances in human inner ear fluid. Inner ear fluid (perilymph and endolymph) was removed from each ear of cadavers, and the ABO group was determined by an absorption technique. The study involved eighty-nine specimens, fourteen of which turned out to be nonsecretors on the basis of not having ABO substances in the salivary glands. As indicated previously, secretors would be expected to have ABO substances present in their body tissue and fluids. Of the seventy-five cases determined to be secretors, ABO group substances could be determined in seventy-two of them. It is of interest to note that there was complete hemolysis of the blood in nine of the cadavers. All nine turned out to be secretors, and it was possible to determine the ABO blood group in each case from the inner ear fluid.

The Collection of Material as Evidence

The handling of materials on which bloodstains or other body fluids are suspected presents many problems. Often, the law enforcement officer is the first official person to arrive at the scene of a crime. Since personnel from a forensic laboratory may not be readily available or even available at all, it is essential that the officer make as critical an examination of the scene as possible. He may have to resort to a naked-eye selection of material for examination which may contain blood or other biological fluids. Much information, for example, can be derived from the physical characteristics of bloodstains (MacDonnell, 1971).

The handling of material suspected of containing blood or other fluids will vary according to the situation. The Colorado Bureau of Investigation requests that the following procedures be utilized for submitting evidence in which biological specimens or items stained with biological fluid are to be examined:

1. Package all clothing exhibits separately in wrapping paper (never in plastic bags) and seal with tape.
2. Small specimens such as hair, bone fragments, and fingernails are packaged in a "druggist fold" (a rectangular piece of paper folded over twice lengthwise at such an angle that one end can be inserted into the other end).
3. Typing of seminal stains usually requires a sample of both the victim's and suspect's saliva and blood. The saliva may be obtained by allowing the individual to expectorate into a tissue (making certain that he has not eaten or chewed gum within an hour of taking the sample).
4. It is advisable to handle all specimens with rubber gloves or forceps, including the clean tissue used for collecting suspect's and/or victim's saliva.

Identification and Processing of Specimens

Readers who are interested in details of the methodologies employed in the serological identification of specimens may refer to several of the books and papers that are listed at the end of this volume, including: Camps (1968), Culliford (1971), Fiori (1962), Glaister (1962), Grunbaum (1972), Kirk (1969), Pereira (1967), Polson (1965), and Sussman (1968).

Once specimens have arrived in the laboratory, three important tasks remain to be accomplished. These tasks first determine the nature of the stain—is it blood, semen, etc.? If the specimen is determined to be blood, it is then necessary to ascertain the animal from which it came. In some cases, if the specimen turns out to be nonhuman, it may not be necessary to proceed further. In other cases, it may be important to determine exactly which nonhuman species left the stain. If the stain is shown to be of human origin, it then remains to carry out whatever blood grouping and typing tests are feasible and important based upon the circumstances surrounding the case, quantity and quality of evidence, and other factors.

A number of tests are available for the identification of bloodstains. An ideal test is one that would be specific for blood. Of the methods that have been utilized, chemical tests have found the greatest application. Two of the most widely used tests are the benzidene test and the phenolphthalein test. Both of these tests are nonspecific, but both have the advantage of being relatively sensitive, the phenolphthalein test having a sensitivity in the range of detecting one part of blood diluted 1 to 5 million times and the benzidene test having a sensitivity of 1 : 200,000 to 1 : 500,000. Both tests are based on the principle of detecting hemoglobin and/or its derivatives, hemoglobin representing one of the characteristic constituents of blood.

Assuming that one of the above tests demonstrates that material in a stain is blood, it may then be necessary to prove that it is human blood (or if not human, at least in some cases, the animal of origin). The test that is used for this purpose is the precipitin test. This test stems from the observation that when human blood is injected into a rabbit, the rabbit responds by making in its blood an antibody which is specific against the human blood. The antihuman rabbit serum will react when it is mixed with other human blood. It should not react with the blood of other animals since it is specific for human blood. It is possible, however, that it might react with the blood of other primates (a fact which demonstrates the serological and evolutionary closeness of man and other primates). In geographical locations or situations where primate blood is likely to be a possible source, it may be necessary to have specific antisera available for some other primates in addition to man.

When human blood is mixed with the antihuman rabbit serum, the precipitin reaction takes place. The latter results in the mixture becoming cloudy through the formation of a white precipitate at the interface between the antihuman serum and the extract. If there is no precipitin reaction, the results indicate that the blood must have originated from some nonprimate mammal. Antisera for some of the common domestic animals such as the cow, pig, dog, etc., are available commercially, and it may even be possible to obtain antisera to some of the common game animals such as deer, elk, etc. The precipitin test is also specific for other human tissues, including bone, flesh, and seminal fluid.

Identification of Blood Type

After a stain has been identified as human blood, it remains for typing tests to be carried out on the samples of blood from the victim and the possible suspect(s) in order to clarify the person of origin of the stain. Until relatively recently, blood grouping tests of stains were limited in routine practice to typing of the ABO system. In some situations, the quantity of blood in the sample may be so small as to preclude testing of many systems. It should be borne in mind that the prospects of excluding an innocent party on the ABO system alone are about one in seven or, as some maintain, one in six. With only a limited amount of sample, careful thought should be given to the tests that are to be run rather than jumping necessarily to the ABO grouping tests first.

Early ABO grouping tests of bloodstains utilized the classical inhibition test. The test was reliable, but it required a relatively large amount of sample. Other tests have been developed which require less material and are equally if not more reliable than the inhibition test. Coombs and Dodd (1961) developed an indirect method which employs an inhibition technique whereby a small portion of the stain is exposed to dilution of antisera and titered to demonstrate a reduction in antibody reactivity.

An absorption-elution method also has been developed and modified for blood-typing of stains. Absorption-elution differs from mixed agglutination in that, after washing away unabsorbed serum, absorbed antibody is eluted from the corpuscular debris by raising the temperature to 50 to 56° C and the eluate is tested with indicator cells. Where absorption and subsequent elution of antibody has occurred, the cells are agglutinated.

Whichever test is employed for typing bloodstains, it is essential that control tests also be run on portions of the unstained cloth, fibers, etc.

In addition to the identification of ABO types in bloodstains, other blood group systems also have been identified, although they have not yet received widespread utilization in a medicolegal sense. Successful identification of the MN blood groups in dried bloodstains was reported by Pereira (1963) who utilized an absorption-elution technique.

Jones and Diamond (1955) have been able to identify the Kell factor in bloodstains using an inhibition procedure. Progress also has been made in the identification of rhesus antigens using a method of absorption-elution. Determination of the Rh phenotype varies with the selection of antisera used and the condition of the stain.

Recent and current research has also been expanded to include the study of serum protein groups, hemoglobin variants, and blood enzyme groups. Most of these groups are identified electrophoretically, and some of them can be reliably identified in dried bloodstains. The excellent treatise by Culliford (1971) offers a useful and practical basis from which a forensic scientist may make a reasonable start in the field of typing of bloodstains in the laboratory. Identification of the Gm groups (Nielsen and Henningsen, 1963) and haptoglobin types appears especially useful in bloodstains (Culliford and Wraxall, 1966). Since the frequencies of variants of the Gm groups and haptoglobin types also vary in the population, use of these systems may be extremely useful in narrowing down the frequencies of blood group combinations when used in combination with other groups such as ABO, MN, Rh, etc.

Determination of Blood Groups in Other Tissues and Biological Fluids

In addition to their determination in blood and bloodstains, certain blood group systems also can be identified in a number of other tissues and biological fluids. As was discussed earlier, about 80 percent of individuals have a gene, the secretor gene, which allows them to secrete the A, B, and AB groups substances in other body fluids. The other 20 percent of individuals are homozygous for the recessive nonsecretor gene and do not secrete these substances in their body fluids. It is of interest to note that the concentration of blood group substances may actually be higher in some of the other fluids than in the blood.

ABO group substances thus have been identified in semen, saliva, hair, nails, and bone. Dodd (1972) has summarized the advances in the typing of bloodstains between the years 1961 and 1970 (Table XI). The more recently developed techniques have the advantage of being more sensitive than the inhibition techniques that had been employed prior to 1961. These tests also can be performed on smaller amounts of test material, so that micromethods have been developed for typing of single fibers and hairs.

TABLE XI

APLICATION OF TECHNIQUES IN TYPING OF BLOODSTAINS*

Year	Development
Pre-1961	Classical inhibition technique for ABO, Rh (D), K, Fy[a]
1961	Mixed agglutination test for ABO
1962	Elution test for ABO
1963	Identification of MN
1963	Identification of GM[a]
1964	Subgrouping of A_1 A_2
1966	Identification of haptoglobin types
1967	Identification of phosphoglucomutase types
1967	Extension of tests for rhesus antigens (Rh-DCEcC[we])
1968	Identification of adenylate kinase
1968	Identification of S groups

* From Dodd (1972).

It has been pointed out earlier that it often is advantageous to be able to type individuals for several blood group systems since it may increase the precision of individual indentification. Dodd (1972) described a case which demonstrates the advantage of the ability to test for several systems in a bloodstain. Two families accused a third of kidnapping a child from each of them. The incident had occurred in Jordan, and blood samples of the six adults and two infants were sent to Dodd in England in the form of heavy bloodstains, each about the size of a postage stamp. The results of typing the stains for ABO, MN, S, D, C, E, c, and phosphoglucomutase showed that it was impossible for the accused couple (F_1M_1) to be the parents of either of the two infants, since they were both S negative and the children, being S positive, had to inherit the S gene from one or other parent. The ABO, MN, and phosphoglucomutase results were not helpful, but the boy was excluded from being the child of F_1 in results obtained with the Rh antigens C and c.

The ABO system supported the claim by the couple F_2M_2 that the boy was theirs and the claim by couple F_3M_3 that they were the parents of the girl.

Little work has been accomplished on the effects of age and material on the identification of bloodstains. Haseeb (1972) tested five samples of bloodstains that had been collected on small pieces of calico. The stains were tested on the third day after collection, then ten years later, and then again twelve years later. The tests that Haseeb performed on the stains included many of the standard tests that a forensic serological laboratory might be expected to perform. They included the benzidine test, which was mentioned earlier as a preliminary screening test for blood; Takayama's hemochromogen test, which is a reliable and sensitive test for blood and which produces crystals of reduced alkaline hematin if the stain is blood; spectroscopic examination, which will confirm if the crystals have been derived from hemoglobin; the precipitin test, which is used for the differentiation of species; and tests for blood grouping by means of the detection of agglutinin.

Although the stains became darker with time and their solubility in saline was decreased, no differences were detected in the results of the tests carried out on the stain on the three occasions.

Rothwell (1970) studied the loss of activity of phosphoglucomutase and adenylate kinase enzymes in blood samples and bloodstains over time. He found that both enzymes could not be grouped indefinitely in bloodstains, with the PGM enzyme being less stable than the AK enzyme.

It is evident that further work is needed to establish the effects of time, types of fabrics, and the mode of preservation on bloodstains.

Bone

Since the early successful blood type determinations of Egyptian mummies by Candela (1936, 1937, 1939, 1940) using an absorption technique, bone blood-grouping has been utilized widely in anthropology and archeology and has found a limited but highly useful application in forensic science. There is some disagreement in the literature about the reliability of typing aged bone. Thieme and Otten (1957) found variable results when testing cadaveral bone that had been typed for its ABO blood groups prior to being buried for a period of less than three years and then being retyped. Of nineteen samples of human bone that had been buried two years in sandy soil, 47 percent were typed incorrectly when tested.

Other workers indicate, however, good success when dealing with bone of "archeological" age. Heglar (1972) has reviewed the history of bone blood-grouping and has provided examples of some of the techniques that he has applied to his archeological studies.

The basic techniques that are used for the determination of blood groups in bone are similar to those used in blood group identification of dried bloodstains. Preliminary titration of the test sera is important, since bone has a relatively high degree of nonspecific adsorptive power and results may lead to a false A or B interpretation. Additional sources of contamination may result from the nonspecific adsorption of plant and animal sources at the site where the bones are found. Heglar's study (1972) approached this problem by typing bone powder against parallel tests of the burial soils. In his study of bone, 10,000 to 30,000 years old, from Borneo, he found that 85 percent of the bone samples could be typed for ABO blood group substances but that the substances were not found in the parallel soil samples.

It is evident that a vital need exists for more basic research on the effects of aging, environmental factors, and sources of contamination on the typing of blood groups in bone. It is necessary to know the nature and the causes of changes in bone tissue that occur under different environmental conditions over time.

Seminal Stains

Persons who possess the secretor gene (Se) also secrete their ABO blood group substances in other body fluids, including semen. Sato and Ottensooser (1967) demonstrated that semen actually contains more blood group substances than saliva. They also reported that semen gave clearer reactions then did saliva.

Although it is not quite specific for semen, the acid phosphatase test is the most commonly used test for screening stains suspected of containing semen. The enzyme acid phosphatase is part of the secretion produced by the prostate gland of the male and forms a constituent part of the semen. Additional proof of the identification of semen would come through the actual microscopic identification of sperm in the test material.

Sivaram (1970) has described a method for the detection and identification of seminal stains based on a modification of the azo-dye technique for acid phosphatase. The method is suitable for normal, aspermic, and contaminated seminal stains.

Other methods of identification of semen employ basic immunological techniques with the utilization of a serum that is specifically anti-human-semen.

Sato and Ottensooser (1967) have described the absorption-inhibition tests that are used for the identification of the ABO blood group substances in semen.

An example of the application of grouping of semen is provided in a case described by Helpern and Wiener (1961) to identify the assailant in a case of rape. Although the vagina of the

TABLE XII

RESULTS OF INHIBITION TESTS ON SEMINAL STAINS FROM RAPE CASE*

Material Examined	Reagent	Test cells (group)	Undiluted	1:2	1:4	1:8	1:16	1:32	1:64	1:128	Interpretation
Seminal stains on clothing	anti-A	A	++	++	+±	+±	+±	+±	+±	+++	
	anti-B	B2	-	-	-	-	-	-	-	+	Group B
	anti-H	H	-	-	-	-	++	++	++	+±	
Controls											
Saliva of nonsecretor	anti-A	A	++	++	+±	+++	+++	+++	+++	+++	
	anti-B	B2	+±	+++	+++	+++	+++	+++	+++	+++	
	anti-H	O	+±	+++	+++	+++	+++	+++	+++	+++	
Commercial A-B-O group substance	anti-A	A	-	-	-	-	-	-	tr.	+	
	anti-B	B2	-	-	tr.	+	++	+±	+±	+±	
	anti-H	O	-	-	-	-	-	-	+±	+	

*From Helpern and Wiener (1961).

victim contained sperm, there was not sufficient semen present to carry out an adequate ABO grouping test. There was, however, a sufficiently large seminal stain present on the victim's clothing. The stain was then used in an inhibition test. A portion of the data of Helpern and Wiener is shown in Table XII. The rape victim belonged to Group O. Results of the grouping of the stain indicated that it must have come from a person belonging to Group B. The authors pointed out that in this particular case, a person was excluded as a suspect because he belonged to Group O.

Fingernails and Hair

Considerable progress has been made in recent years in the determination of blood groups from hair, eyebrows, and fingernails. Although these substances possess only low amounts of the blood group substances, they offer some key advantages to forensic science in that they are easy to collect and preserve.

Both elution methods (Yada, Okane, and Sano, 1966a, b, c, d) and mixed agglutination methods (Lincoln and Dodd, 1968) have been employed in blood group determinations of hair. Yada and his associates have been successful in determining ABO blood group antigens using the elution technique on even a single piece of scalp hair, pubic hair, or axillary hair as well as eyebrows, eyelashes, and the vibrissae in the nostrils.

Table XIII presents the results of Yada et al. (1966d) of the elution tests performed on eyebrows, eyelashes, and vibrissae as

TABLE XIII

ABO TYPING OF EYEBROWS, EYELASHES,
VIBRISSAE, AND EPIDERMIS*

Eluate From Eyebrow		Eluate From Eyelash		Eluate From Vibrissa		Eluate From Epidermis		Inferred Blood Group	Known Blood Group
+A	+B	+A	+B	+A	+B	+A	+B		
−	−	−	+	−	−	/	/	O	O
+	−	/	/	+	−	/	/	A	A
+	−	/	/	+	−	/	/	A	A
+	+	+	+	+	+	/	/	AB	AB

* From Yada, Okane, Sado, and Fukumori (1966).

well as on epidermal fragments. In a number of cases, the blood groups of the corpses from which the specimens were taken were unknown, and blood grouping of a small piece of skin of the abdomen also was done. Results demonstrated that all the hair specimens derived from a single individual showed uniformity in the reactions to anti-A and anti-B sera, and the blood groups determined on the hair were in complete concord with the known blood groups or with those determined on the epidermal fragments, indicating the high reliability of the techniques employed.

Outteridge (1963) also has utilized successfully the absorption-elution method for the determination of ABO group from fingernails. Nail fragments do not react as strongly as similar weights of blood, and it may be necessary therefore to use longer periods of absorption than with other substances.

CHAPTER 9

Handwriting

I**T IS LIKELY** that soon after writing was developed, man began to wonder about the possibility of determining something about the identity and personality of an individual through his handwriting. Even as early as 1622, Camillo Baldi, a physician, had published a book entitled *The Means of Knowing the Habits and Qualities of a Writer from His Letters.* Today, the tremendous interest in handwriting is reflected in the numerous courses that have sprung up in cities and campuses throughout the country to inform people about the art and science of handwriting analysis. Unfortunately, handwriting interpretation often is associated by the scientist and the lay person alike with

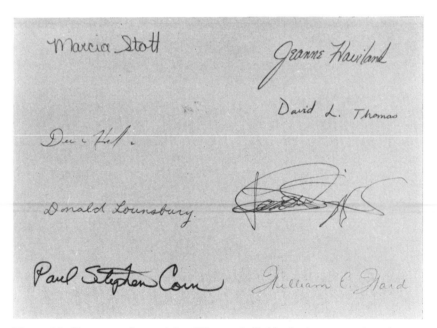

Figure 35. Signatures from eight different individuals demonstrating the tremendous diversity of handwriting. The ease of someone copying these signatures also would vary greatly.

124

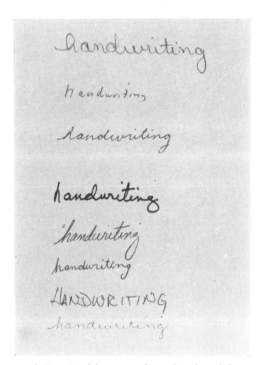

Figure 36. The word *Handwriting* as written by the eight persons who provided the signatures in Figure 35. It is of interest to note that two of the eight individuals in this sample use a modified form of printing.

circuses, carnival booths, witchcraft, practitioners of the occult, and fortune tellers. These types of associations no doubt have hindered and continue to hinder scientific endeavors in the field.

As with other methods of individual identification, some notable mistakes have been made. Perhaps the most famous case of them all was the Dreyfus case. Alfred Dreyfus was a captain in the French army who was accused and convicted in 1894 by a military court of transmitting secrets to a foreign power. One of the main pieces of evidence against Dreyfus was a document supposedly written by him. The head of the French Identification Service at that time was Alphose Bertillon, one of the early pioneers in forensic science. Although Bertillon was not a "handwriting expert," he regarded himself as one and testified that the handwriting sample in the document did in fact belong to Dreyfus. The testimony coming from such a well-known and well-respected person as Bertillon aided in convicting Dreyfus. It should be noted that other testimony from qualified document examiners reported that the document in question could not have been written by Dreyfus.

The original trial, retrial, and final pardon make for an interesting bit of judicial history. Following the trial in 1894, Dreyfus was sentenced to life imprisonment in Devils' Island. He was retried in 1899 and was once again found guilty. He eventually was pardoned by President Loubet, and the supreme court of France finally exonerated him completely in 1906.

Basic Terminology

Baxter (1966) has discussed the definitions and implications of such terms as handwriting, graphology, handwriting expert, and questioned document examiners. It is necessary to keep some of these distinctions in mind. Handwriting is a kind or style of writing, a system of communicating by means of certain symbolic forms.

Graphology is the study of handwriting, especially in relation to the author's character. A "graphologist" thus tries to infer something about the character and personality of an individual from the handwriting of that individual. The science of graphoanalysis has a history that traces back more than fifty years, and there is considerable interest in the science today.

A "handwriting expert" also is someone who makes a detailed study of handwriting. However, the handwriting expert usually has the task of trying to determine the author of a piece of writing or whether or not two specimens of writing were made by the same individual.

Naftali (1965) has described succinctly the work of the handwriting expert:

> In handwriting identification, the expert is called upon to identify a person by comparing recordings of movement, that is to say, by inference. His task is not performed through comparing and calculating fixed characteristics as is done in the objective method. It is also not the subjective form of direct identification based on memory traces of fixed characteristics. In a way the handwriting expert may be compared

to a witness identifying a person well known to him by his gait, posture, or other frequently perceived complex movement patterns without seeing his face. For the handwriting expert does just this: He compares traces of purposeful motor behavior recorded in conventional symbols with a writing instrument in various situations. . . . Thus the task of the document examiner is somewhat similar to that of an art critic trying to establish authorship of a painting by getting familiar with other works of the same painter. All considerations regarding period, style, mannerism, content, means of expression, wilful changes, or forgeries, so important in the evaluation of creative arts, are prominent in the process of judging a piece of writing. To get at the causes of the subjective certainty of an examiner of Q.D. (questioned documents) and also at the source of possible errors of judgment, the *mental process* involved in *comparing visual images* must be studied.

It may be noted in the above passage that Naftali has used the terms *handwriting expert* and *document examiner* interchangeably. However, the questioned document examiner typically has duties that extend far beyond those of someone who is just a handwriting expert. Thus, the questioned document examiner may be concerned not only with the comparison and identification of handwriting specimens but also may be concerned with the means by which the writing is accomplished. He may be interested in the instruments of writing—pencils, pens, brushes, machines, etc. He might examine the medium on which the writing was produced—the type of paper, parchment, etc. What type of substance was used? This would lead to the identification of various fluids, including inks, paints, dyes, etc. As Baxter (1966) points out, even the punched cards, patterns, or tapes of the modern computing machines could be the subject of questioned document examinations.

Seals or impressions of wax, plastic, and ductile metals are also examined in the questioned documents laboratory to determine whether or not they are genuine and/or are in their original (applied) state. Alterations, by addition or erasure, to the "written" material content of a document form a large part of the questioned document examiner's duties, as does the search for evidence of interference to documents by way of opening and refastening the covers of packets, letters, etc.

Given the vast and varied potential duties of a questioned documents examiner, one may wonder what training and background would be required for such a person. In England, in 1964, a Questioned Document Sub-Section of the British Academy of Forensic Sciences was formed. At that time, it was felt that the following basic educational requirements should be met: "At least two subjects in the General Certificate of Education (Advanced Level) from the following: Chemistry and Physics or Mathematics or Biology. Coupled to these subjects, and for specific study, should be such related subjects as: Ink and Paper Making, Printing, Photography, Microscopy, Writing Instruments (including Typewriters)."

The American Academy of Forensic Sciences also has a Questioned Documents Section.

Graphoanalysis

Psychologists and psychiatrists are making increasing use of graphoanalysis in individual identification and in the determination of personality characteristics. Through a detailed examination of a person's handwriting it often is possible for a trained analyst to identify many different mental and physical traits of that person.

The literature of studies examining the relationship between personality and handwriting is extensive, and results from different studies often are contradictory. Some studies have yielded essentially negative results and others, to some extent, positive results.

One of the first scientific studies was carried out by Hull and Montgomery (1919), who studied the relationship between handwriting and personality characteristics. They utilized six personality traits and determined the rank order correlation between the rankings of the subjects, as determined from the frequency of the signs in their handwriting (as defined by graphologists) and the rankings of the subjects by their fraternity brothers based on the same personality traits. Hull and Montgomery were unable to find any significant relationships between handwriting and the personality traits.

An interesting study was performed by Pascal and Suttell

(1947). A graphologist had indicated that she could distinguish normal and psychotic persons solely on the basis of samples of their handwriting. However, upon testing the graphologist under controlled conditions, Pascal and Suttell found that the woman could not distinguish handwriting samples of normal and psychotic persons with any degree of success. Her accuracy, in fact, was no greater than would have been expected under chance decision making.

The far-reaching claims made by many graphologists have tended to mask some of the positive findings that have been reported. One of the leading workers in the field has been H. J. Eysenck, who has done extensive work in the overall area of abnormal and normal behavior. A study reported in 1945 compared the results of graphoanalysis of psychiatric hospital patients with results from their psychiatric examinations. Information about the patients was provided concerning their case histories, intelligence test scores, clinical description of their personalities by psychiatrists, and the results of a forced choice personality questionnaire. Based only on his knowledge of the subject gained through an analysis of the handwriting, the graphologist estimated the subject's level of intelligence and attempted to match the handwriting to the personality description. Results indicated that the graphologist did not estimate the intelligence level of the subject successfully but did match the handwriting with the clinical personality description with some success. The forced choice personality questionnaire also yielded interesting results. The graphologist filled out the personality questionnaire, basing his answers on the personality of the subject as perceived in the handwriting. It was found that the questionnaire was answered by the graphologist with better than merely chance accuracy.

In an additional study, Eysenck (1948) determined that a graphologist was not able to differentiate different levels of neurosis among hospital patients who had been diagnosed as neurotics. The graphologist, however, did far better in the agreement of ratings on the neurotocism scale, based on handwriting samples and ratings of the same patients, who had been given battery of tests which measured the neurotocism factor. A significant correlation was obtained between the two types of ratings. The positive findings led Eysenck to conclude that a person's handwriting may reveal something about personality traits.

Faust and Price (1972) carried out an interesting study utilizing twins in order to obtain an objective assessment of the validity of trying to use handwriting to determine personality attributes. They tested twenty-four pairs of identical and nonidentical twins. Twins have been utilized extensively in biomedical research. The use of twins overcomes many of the disadvantages that are usually present when studying human populations. The twin pairs can be matched for age, sex, social class, and other environmental variables associated with family background, including schooling. The latter is particularly important when analyzing handwriting. Since the twins have been raised in the same home, the parents are able to furnish reliable ratings of the twins' personalities.

Personality scores were obtained for each subject, and each pair of twins was rated by their parents on a questionnaire comparing their personality and development. These ratings were compared with ratings of within-pair personality differences based on the examination of samples of handwriting by a consultant graphologist and by a team of eight mental health professionals. The latter were "amateurs" regarding graphoanalysis.

In brief, the authors concluded that handwriting is not likely to be helpful in the study of neuroticism. However, there was some evidence that handwriting was somewhat useful in the ratings related to extraversion.

Faust and Price attempted to ascertain which features of the handwriting were used by the raters. The following items were measured: (1) the number of words in the first five lines; (2) the height of the first five lines; (3) the slope, in degrees, of the fifth line; (4) the slope, in degrees, of the first letter containing an upright stroke; and (5) the height of the letter M in an expression beginning "My dear. . . ." The slope of the letters and the number of words seemed to be important features in influencing the handwriting ratings.

Graphoanalysis has found some medical applications in such

problems as migraine and homosexuality (Holt, 1965) and schizophrenia (Rosenthal, 1963). In his book *The Genain Quadruplets,* Rosenthal reported on the developmental history of schizophrenia in identical female quadruplets. Handwriting samples of the girls as high-school students (ages sixteen to seventeen) were available and again as hospital patients (ages twenty-eight to twenty-nine). A graphologist was able to match successfully the earlier and later samples. Additional studies in this area would be most useful, as it might be possible to study the premorbid personality of patients who subsequently develop some psychiatric disorder.

"Trained" vs "Untrained" Graphologists

Although there still may be some questions concerning the overall capacities of graphologists to assess personality characteristics, there is no doubt that someone who is trained and experienced in handwriting analysis performs much better than an untrained person. Some of the early studies utilized only untrained judges and do not allow for a direct comparison of trained versus untrained judges. Nevertheless, results of such studies may shed some light on the importance of training in graphoanalysis. Middleton (1941a), for example, studied a group of seventy-six students who were untrained in graphology. The students had to analyze the handwriting of subjects and rate them according to their levels of self-confidence, sociability, and neuroticism. The ratings based only on handwriting were then compared to ratings of the subjects determined from their scores for the same traits on the Bernreuter Personality Inventory. A significant but low correlation was observed for neuroticism, but the correlations for self-confidence and sociability were not significant. The results indicated that untrained persons cannot judge these personality attributes with any degree of accuracy.

Various workers, including Bloom and Basinger (1932), Middleton (1941b), and Secord (1949), have demonstrated that untrained judges are not able to judge the intelligence of subjects from their handwriting with greater than chance accuracy.

In a study reported by Castelnuovo-Tedesco (1946), untrained judges were able to judge the sex of the subjects correctly in 66 percent of the cases. Six judges rated a group of subjects for intelligence, anxiety, and compulsiveness. Contingency coefficients of .60, .33, and .27 were obtained respectively. Higher coefficients were obtained after the judges had received some training in graphology. The coefficients rise to .64, .41, and .32 following training.

Some interesting applications of graphology have been made by industrial firms. Sonnermann and Kernan (1962) compared the ratings given executives of a large corporation by their superiors and two sets of ratings by a graphologist predicting their performance from their handwriting. The first set of ratings was based upon the analyses of a sample of handwriting written at the time the subject was hired, and the second was based upon a handwriting sample written within six months of the date of analysis. The subjects were rated on idea ability, executive caliber, expression, achievement, and overall value to the company. The correlations obtained ranged from .36 to .48 for each scale and were all significant at the .05 level or above. The reliabilities of the graphologists' ratings ranged from .64 to .85 (based on the correlation between the ratings obtained from each of the two samples of handwriting for each subject). Sonnemann and Kernan concluded that blind graphological evaluations were significantly related to performance on the job.

J. F. McCarthy (1976) has provided an interesting and useful informal summary of his thoughts and experiences concerning handwriting and behavior:

1. Beauty is a quality seldom heard in other forensic sciences. Some handwriting may be classified as beautiful. In fact, the word "calligraphy" means the art of beautiful writing.

2. Handwriting most certainly reflects some aspect of the writer's personality. And that is about all you can say with assurance on a subject which has been remarkedly blessed with numerous theoretical insights of dubious value.

3. Handwriting is in essence nothing more than a form of visual behavior, graphically recorded and relatively permanent. It is the result of the writer's physiological, psychological, and environmental life.

4. In observing and commenting on the behavior of another person, we can only say how he normally behaves. We can never say that he is utterly incapable of another form of behavior. Thus, in handwriting cases, identifying the author of a writing is easier than the process of elimination. Nevertheless, eliminations can be made when a reasonable and prudent examiner finds that any other explanation of a large number of dissimilarities are so glaring that it would require tremendous intellectual gymnastics to come to any other conclusion.

5. Since behavior at a particular time in a particular set of circumstances is unpredictable, it is extremely difficult to eliminate as suspects those individuals whose writing reflects about the same skill as that found on the questioned document, even though other characteristics are completely different.

6. An habitual action tends to become automatic, that is, to take place independently of attention. Few people can tell which shoe they put on first in the morning because the act is so habitual as to require no attention. Handwriting of the skilled writer is acquired through practice. The practice is continued until the exact movements can be executed unconsciously. When consciousness is applied to an activity which has become automatic the interference may become disastrous. This is an important point to keep in mind when examining "request" writings, since in executing specimens the subject usually becomes aware that his handwriting contains identifying characteristics. As the result of this awareness even the most cooperative subject may introduce some rare characteristics in his writing and the uncooperative subject's writing may be entirely unnatural.

7. The unconscious nature of habit is a significant psychological fact. It means that our particular handwriting is motivated by factors of which we are unaware and which we are unable to recall.

8. The act of writing is a semiautomatic act somewhat like the act of breathing. It is normally carried out without conscious thought, but it can be altered. For example, one can hold one's breath, one can voluntarily change the breathing pattern over a short period, but over the long run one's attention is directed to some other thought. It is important in collecting request writings

to divert the attention of the writer on numerous occasions and in as many as practicable.

9. One does not outgrow handwriting habits. The tendency is to grow into them.

10. Can examiners use their present results to predict what will happen in the future (that is, how a person will write on the next occasion)? Since behavior can be modified at any time, we cannot predict that an individual will continue to act in the same way. For example, a confirmed smoker may give up cigarettes or a nonsmoker may take them up. However, normally, a whole group of unassociated habits is not changed. For example, stopping smoking and changing the shoe put on first in the morning are unrelated. Thus, while a person may change his writing habits, he can be expected to keep his habits of arranging material on paper.

11. In attempting disguise the writer can be expected to revert to an earlier form of behavior, that is, re-adopt a letter formation previously used. Thus, in examinations involving possible disguise in a questioned writing it may be wise to look for samples written years earlier. This is particularly noticeable when capital letters are dramatically different.

12. In fatigue conditions the writer must resort more and more to habit in writing, and normal characteristics reappear even when he is attempting disguise. This is also true of rapid writing.

13. In a specific situation a person is prone to do what he has done in that specific situation before. In psychology, this is called "propensity." Thus, in cases where the forger's name and the name being forged have some common letters, one may find that at the end of one series of letters, another has been formed, in whole or in part, which reflects a letter found in the forger's name.

14. Introjection is a mode of embracing the personality elements that are admired in other persons. It may be thought of as the taking for one's own the feelings, attitudes, standards, restrictions, prohibitions, physical gestures, and characteristics of parents or parental figures. Thus, in addition to enjoying a neuromuscular system similar to our parents, brothers, and sis-

ters, we consciously embrace graphic forms which we admire in members of our family as well as teachers, friends, and so forth.

15. Some people deteriorate or change dramatically with the years while others do not. Some writings change with the years and others do not.

16. Moving the pen off the paper permits the attention of the writer to be directed away from the act; thus, more variation can be expected to appear in the writing of numerals and in hand-printing than in cursive writing.

17. One can induce an earlier form of behavior by having a person write with the weaker hand. This is true principally with letter formations, but is probably also true of such as rhythm and line quality.

18. A transitory change in characteristics may be injected into handwriting by temporary physical and mental conditions, such as fatigue, nervous tension, and intoxication or severe illness, from which the writer ultimately recovers. In these cases, hand-writing reverts to its normal qualities after the causes of the deterioration are removed.

19. Writing is a function of the central nervous system. Thus, any substance which affects the central nervous system will affect the writing, for better or worse.

20. One must observe behavior over a period of time. One cannot determine a person's normal behavior based on a single check at one point in an individual's history. Thus, in handwriting examinations and unlike fingerprint identifications, one needs more than a single standard for comparison.

21. Training produces its effects on habit systems without leaving any explicit memories. The automaticity of habit is an important feature in mental economy. However, habit works against us as well as for us and bad habits can become second nature as readily as good ones. Thus, some individuals not only do not remember how they arrange their material on paper, but do not know that these habits of writing might be wrong, or, at least, unusual.

22. Strong emotional stimuli may produce disorganized responses in some individuals. Thus, some subjects in executing re-

quest writing may appear to be intentionally distorting their writing when in fact their erratic writing style is due solely to the inability of the subject to function normally in a stress situation.

23. The melody of a musical score does not depend on the parts but on structure, for the parts may all be changed by transposing to another key, and yet the melody remains intact. The parts have been altered, the whole is still the same. Changing the angle of a writing is nothing more than changing the key. The handwriting is still identifiable.

24. Perseveration is the tendency to repeat or continue an activity. Thus, when an individual starts to write there is a momentum involving inertia which impels him to continue the same habits throughout his life.

25. Practice results in improving any motor skill, thus the flat statement that no one "can write better than his best" is erroneous if there is time and effort available for practice. However, even after the expenditure of time a writer will return towards his norm when the time and effort expire.

Factors Affecting Handwriting

It is evident from the above that a number of physical and biological factors are known which may influence a person's handwriting, either showing up as a temporary deviation from the normal style or else showing up as a permanent change as illustrated by a long-term trend. The emotional state of the writer at any one time may have a profound influence. The posture of the writer, the lighting, the type of paper, the surface on which the writing is done, and the writing instrument all may exert an influence on the quality of handwriting.

Naftali (1965) has proposed five elements which influence writing on the basis of work from the medical or neurophysiological point of view:

1. Inborn movement forms.

    These movements have repetitive rhythmic character and are connected with reflexive and instinctive behaviors. The movements are subject to involuntary changes but cannot be readily changed by wilful or conscious effort.

2. Acquired movement patterns.

Acquired movements are directed, in part, by the higher brain centers of the cerebral cortex. Consideration of our present writing indicates that coordination is necessary for up-and-down movements as well as the forming of the specific letters.

3. Muscular tension.

Pophal (1950) differentiates between two distinct types of tension which are evident in handwriting. The types are *pressure,* which is characterized by the rhythmical alternation of tension and release in the up-and-down strokes, and the *stiffening* tension, which is a static form of "isotonic" muscular contraction.

4. The fourth element refers to the effect of the mental image of the desired writing form which is originally caused by copybook standards and is strongly influenced by changing taste and developmental factors during a person's lifetime.

5. The writing situation.

Situational factors influencing handwriting are common knowledge, but individual adjustment patterns will produce so many different responses to identical stimuli that it is difficult to generalize.

Systems of Classification

Numerous systems have been developed for the classification of handwriting. Size, slant, pressure, form, speed, and spacing are some of the factors that have been used. Smith (1964) described at least 100 additional factors which facilitate the classification of handwriting. He refers to the subdivisions as *determining tendencies* "because though perhaps they are not measurable, they will appear often enough to be called a tendency, and a strong tendency determines the look of a writing." Presumably, an individual's tendencies reflect minor personal habits that have become incorporated into the individual's handwriting.

Examples of some of the tendencies are the subdivisions under *loops,* such as may be found in the letters *y* or *l.* Some of the trends of loops as presented by Smith include the following: enlarged, tall or long, swollen, bloated, greatly exaggerated, reduced to a single line, short, inconsistent in length, regular and balanced in size proportions, omitted altogether, bent way over, very heavy, very light, made in an angular fashion, twisting around other letters, swinging off to the left, and swinging off to the right.

All systems of handwriting classification ultimately aim to find out what is personal and unique about a person's handwriting. The systems are based on the assumption that writing is, for the most part, a process that is a relatively permanent and an unconscious motor activity. In fact, most individuals would have great difficulty trying to describe their own handwriting, and many individuals cannot even recognize their own handwriting.

Baxter (1973) has reviewed many of the classical works that have been used in the classification and measurement of handwriting. These works include books by Hagan (1894), Blackburn and Caddell (1909), Osborn (1929), Harrison (1958), and Bates (1970).

All of the systems have employed the general procedures and principles that have been utilized so successfully in the natural sciences, including botany, geology, and zoology.

Baxter's conclusions, although somewhat pessimistic, reflect the nature of the problems associated with the classification of handwriting:

> All systems, methods, or techniques involving the "classification" and/or "measurement" of handwriting in identification exercises have failed in universal acceptance or adoption. This failure is due, in the main, to the intrinsic variation of handwritten shapes, produced as they are by complex neuromuscular activity, apparently incapable of exact replication. It is the present writer's opinion that there can be little valid optimism for such a radical change in systems design as will eliminate or accommodate this paramount natural fact.

Summary

Most workers are somewhat pessimistic about the overall usefulness of handwriting in problems of identification. Baxter (1973), for example, regards handwriting identification as "probably the most speculative of the forensic disciplines."

The importance of individual expertise and experience is nowhere greater than in the work carried out by the questioned documents examiner. The general conclusions and problems have been summarized well by the late Doctor Kirk (1953):

Handwriting identification, many authorities to the contrary notwithstanding, has yet to be reduced to the precision and objectivity characteristic of most criminalistics testing. Competent document examiners apply to it a keenness of observation characteristic of the scientist, combined with logical reasoning, and an orderly and thorough examination. In addition, there is a very important factor of experience, and even of intuition, not readily reduced to routine, impossible to teach in a definite manner and yet highly critical to the end result.

CHAPTER 10

Hair

HAIR MAY PLAY an important part in the identification of individuals. This is especially true in crimes of violence where physical contact is likely to take place. There often is likely to be an extensive exchange of hair between the victim and the person committing the crime. Hair from the victim may be found on the suspect's clothing or on some other physical object. And, conversely, hair from the suspect may be found on the victim's clothing or on the victim himself. It is obvious that the searching for hairs as evidence may be a most difficult and time-consuming effort. However, the potential significance of hair as evidence cannot be overemphasized. The use of hair evidence may be a great assistance in identifying the weapon or object used in a crime. Hair may even be of assistance in identifying a vehicle involved in a hit-and-run accident.

Scientific interest in the study of hair and its application to forensic science extends back over 100 years. Pfaff, in 1869, wrote a book entitled *Human Hair in Its Physiological, Pathological, and Forensic Significance.* Since that time, an increasing number of biologists and forensic scientists have been involved in trichology, the science or study of hair and its diseases. In addition to its value in individual identification, hair also may serve as an indicator of disease and pathological states (Ferriman, 1971).

A useful summary statement of the nature of the art of the identification of hair is provided by Wildman (1961):

> First, although books and photographs are useful as guides, there is no reliable short-cut method for identifying animal fibres by simply "matching up" the microscopical appearance of an unknown fibre with a photomicrograph; the observer should have had experience in the examination and interpretation of diagnostic features of a variety of fibres. Secondly, and contrary to suggestions made in some publications, no measurement method, such as for example the measurement of distances between successive external scale margins or the measurement of fibre diameter, will itself reveal the precise origin of a fibre.

140

Thirdly, chemical tests do not distinguish between animal fibres, since all animal fibres consist of the same substance, namely keratin. The only satisfactory procedure is to use the method of microscopy with a sound knowledge of fibre morphology and careful interpretation of the observations made.

General Biology of Hair

Hair is a unique feature of mammals, including man. It covers the entire body of most mammals, although in some mammals it may be restricted to a few specific areas or may be almost lacking entirely in marine mammals such as the whale. The human, compared to most mammals, is relatively hairless, a fact which has led to the title of a recent book, *The Naked Ape* (Morris, 1967).

A cross-sectional view of the skin, showing the relationship of a hair and hair follicle to other structures in the skin, is shown in Figure 37. A hair consists of dead epidermal cells and has grown out from living cells in the root of the hair. Involuntary muscles (the *arrector pili*) are associated with each hair follicle near its base. The hairs do not project vertically from the skin but come out at an angle. When the *arrector pili* muscles contract, the hair is brought to an erect position. This gives the well-known effect of "hair standing on end" observed in many animals or "goose flesh" in man.

When viewed in cross section, a typical hair is seen to consist of three layers: the medulla, the cortex, and the cuticle. The medulla is the inner or central shaft of the hair. In humans, this central canal may be continuous, or it may be irregular and interrupted by a series of hollow spaces. The width of the shaft may be fairly uniform or varying, but it usually makes up less of the total hair width in humans than it does in other animals. In some instances, the medulla may be lacking entirely.

The cortex surrounds the medulla and comprises the bulk of the hair; the cuticle is the single outer layer of scales. The color of hair is a result of the amount and distribution of pigments and the actual structure of the hair. Both the medulla and cortex may contain pigments, but the cuticle does not. It has been estimated that the adult human male possesses about 5 million hair follicles. With normal aging, there is a decrease in the num-

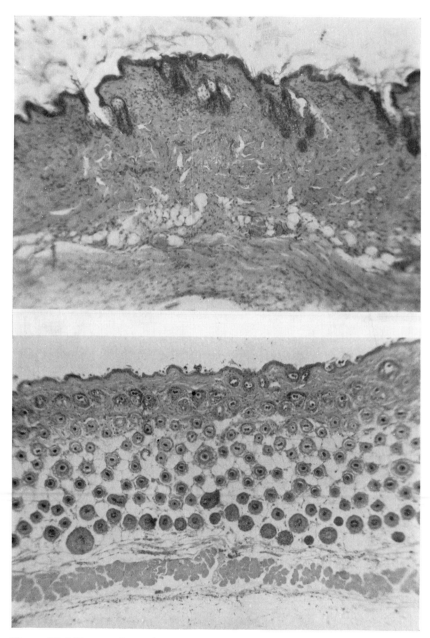

Figure 37. Microscopic sections of mouse skin showing hair follicles in longitudinal sections (above) and tangential sections (below).

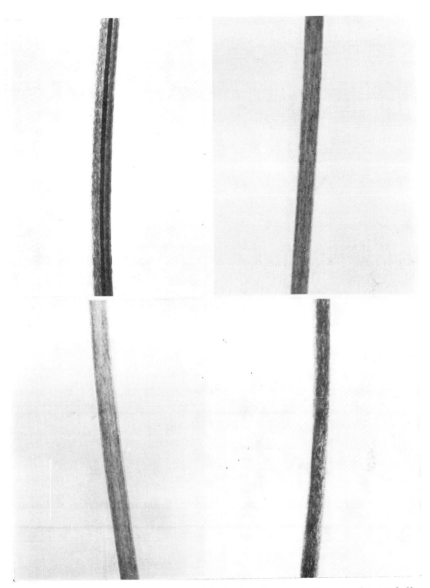

Figure 38. Examples of human head hair showing variations in the medulla: continuous medulla (upper left), fragmented medulla (upper right), no medulla (lower left), dispersed pigmentation (lower right).

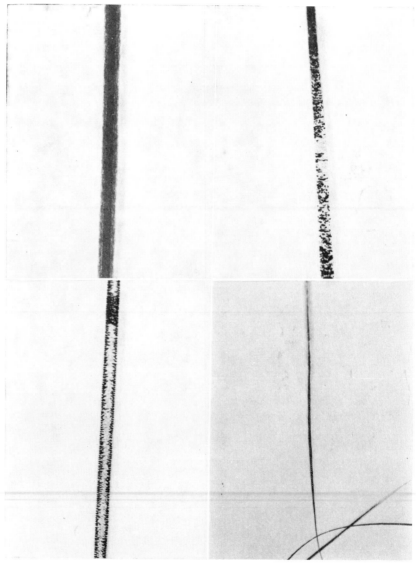

Figure 39. Dorsal guard hairs from the muskrat (upper left), fox (upper right), marmot (lower left), and mole (lower right).

ber of follicles, and the decrease is accentuated in individuals who are going bald. The distribution and amount of body hair may be affected markedly by race as well as by sex.

Garn (1951) has described six morphological types of hair in man as follows: I. Head hair; II. Eyebrow and eyelash hair; III. Beard and moustache hair; IV. Body hair; V. Pubic hair; VI. Axillary hair. The hairs of types I, II, V, and VI show little variation in their patterns and quantities and are of little use in studying differences among the races. The hairs of the body, beard, and moustache show greater variation and are useful for differentiating the races. Hrdy and Baden (1973) studied the biochemical variation of hair in different races of man and in nonhuman primates. They utilized a number of methods of study, including amino acid analysis, acrylamide gel electrophoresis, x-ray diffraction studies, and stress-strain analysis. Their samples included hair from European, Mongolian, African, Melanesian, and Australian persons. Hair of the different races produced identical results, indicating that the variables producing phenotypic differences in human hair forms are probably not on the level of primary or secondary biochemical structure.

Information to Be Derived from Hair Samples

Although a person's hair is not unique to him and by itself cannot furnish conclusive identification, nevertheless, much valuable information may be obtained from a systematic study of hair evidence. In its characteristics of structure, including the presence or absence of a medulla, the features of the medulla, the patterns of scales on the surface, and other characteristics, human hair can be distinguished from other animals, including even those primates with the closest physical resemblance to man. Differences among different racial groups of people may be discerned on the basis of the morphological characteristics of the hair. In the same individual, it may even be possible to determine the region of the body from which the hair originated.

Is the Sample Actually Hair?

Although the above question may seem to be an overly simple one, it nevertheless is a very basic and essential one. There are many types of fibers which superficially bear a close resemblance to animal (including human) hair. Fibers may trace back to plant (linen, cotton, etc.), mineral (asbestos, glass, etc.), or synthetic (nylon, rayon, etc.) origin. Microscopic examination should readily distinguish hair from the above types of fibers. As discussed above, hair has a characteristic and distinctive structure consisting of a medulla, cortex, and cuticle. If the specimen in question does not exhibit such characteristics, it most likely is not hair and can be considered to be a fiber of some sort. It is beyond the scope of this book to discuss the significance of fiber identification in forensic science. Suffice it to say that detailed morphological and chemical examination of fibers may also yield valuable information related to identification. Fibers from an individual piece of clothing may be as unique as many other attributes of the individual. In some cases, it may be possible to match torn fibers and threads with the object from which they came.

If the sample in question is hair, what kind of hair is it? Is it human or nonhuman?

It is usually relatively easy to differentiate human hair from hair of other animals. Niyogi (1962) mentions seven characteristic features of the human hair:

1. A thin medullary canal, and its absence in some hair.
2. A broad cortex.
3. Cuticular scales which are less projecting and which show a great deal of overlapping. The cuticular margins are even.
4. A medullary index below 0.30

$$\left(\text{medullary index} = \frac{\text{the diameter of the medulla}}{\text{the diameter of the whole shaft}} \right)$$

In nonhuman animals, the medullary index usually is above 0.50.

5. Cross sections which are almost circular or oval in shape.
6. The pigment granules of the cortex are distributed towards the periphery.
7. The presence of short and broad scales (Scale Type VII—

irregular annular), according to the classification of Moritz (1939).

In some cases, it may be necessary to use most, if not all, of these features in order to affix a positive determination of human on the sample in question, since some animal hairs may share some of these features with human hairs. As might be expected, animals that are more closely related in a biological or evolutionary sense tend to have more similar hairs than do less related animals. For example, hairs of the higher primates, including the gorilla and the chimpanzee, also have a low medullary index and in general are quite similar to those of the human. However, the human medulla is still smaller than that of the gorilla or the chimpanzee. In addition, there are differences in the distribution of pigment granules in the cortex and in the scales. In addition to having a collection of representative human hairs, an active forensic trichology laboratory also should maintain a representative collection of animal hairs.

If the hair is not human, from what animal did it come?

Assuming the sample in question has been identified as not being from a human, in some cases no further differentiation may be necessary to try to pinpoint from what animal the hair did originate. Applications of this sort, however, may be of considerable value in cases involving violations of hunting laws.

A number of excellent publications exist concerning the identification of animal hair, including Hausman (1920, 1924, 1930), Mathiak (1938), Mayer (1952), Stains (1958), Spence (1963), Wildman (1961), and Williams (1938). Identification of animal hair is based upon the same general characteristics discussed above, i.e. the character of the medulla, the amount and distribution of pigments, the type of cuticular scale patterns, and hair size. In many cases, it is possible to identify hair down to the species from which it came. Spence (1963) and Stains (1958) reported 78 percent and 85 percent accuracy, respectively, in the utilization of their keys for the identification of "unknown" hairs.

What Other Information May Be Derived from the Hair?

Given that a sample of hair is human hair, it may be possible to derive other information as to the part of the body it came from and the age, sex, and race of the person who left the hair.

Region of the Body

As indicated earlier, hairs from different regions of the body do differ from each other. The six types of hair recognized by Garn (1951) are differentiated on the basis of length and other characteristics. Head hair is 100 to 1000 mm in length and 25 to 125 mm in cross-sectional diameter. The hairs have a relatively small root, a tapered tip, and are usually medullated. Hairs of the eyebrows and eyelashes are about 100 mm long and are curved, coarse, smooth with a punctate tip, and possess a large medulla. Beard and moustache hairs range in size from 50 to 300 mm and have a larger root, blunter tip, and a more irregular structure than other head hair. Body hair is 3 to 60 mm in length and has a long tip and irregularities in structure. Pubic hair is 10 to 60 mm in length and is somewhat coarse and irregular and asymmetrical in cross section, with many constrictions and twists. Axillary hair is 10 to 50 mm in length. The hairs are coarse with a blunt tip and are usually abraded and split, with many cortical fusi.

Sex

It is usually not possible to tell with any degree of certainty the sex of an individual from a hair sample. With the present hair styles, it has become even more difficult. In the past, men usually had much shorter hair than women, did not brush or comb it as much, and only rarely did they treat it with dyes, tints, or bleaches. Nowadays, the sex differences in hairstyles are no longer nearly as prevalent. There are, however, some significant differences which may be of value in exceptional cases. In general, the scalp hair of the male has a larger diameter than that of the female and tends to be more wiry. Male eyebrows are thinner and more wiry than those of females.

Several minor differences are found between male and female pubic hairs. These differences may be of some value in sexual assault cases. The pubic hairs of males typically have thick roots and are thin compared to female pubic hairs which have thin roots and are thicker.

Greenwell et al. (1941) declared that the refractive index appeared to be one of the best criteria for the determination of sex and pointed out that a relatively large difference existed between male and female hair of Caucasian origin.

According to Frankenberg (1959), the frequency of sex chromatin positive cells in the male is 3 to 5 percent, compared to 30 to 61 percent in the female.

Age

Age also is a feature which cannot be readily determined in hair. Although, in general, gray or white hair tends to be more common in older persons, there are many cases of hairs without any pigment in young persons. Oesterlen (1935) felt that the diameter of the hair was related to the age of the person. From a value of 0.024 mm shortly after birth, the diameter increased to 0.053 mm at fifteen years of age, and to 0.07 mm in adults.

Race

Among the major races of man there are some striking differences in hair morphology. The amount of pigment varies widely, being quite dense in Mongolians and Negroes. The pigment among the hairs of Mongolians tends to have a much more even and regular distribution than in Negroes, where the distribution is much more irregular. The cross-sectional shape of the hair also varies. Mongolian hair is nearly cylindrical, Caucasian hair is of an oval shape, and hair of Negroes is flattened and ellipsoid in shape.

As Hrdy (1973) has noted, "Cranial hair form has been one of the major racial criteria since the beginning of anthropological thought." Surprisingly, little systematic research has been carried out to examine populational differences in hair form. In his recent work, Hrdy studied eight hair form variables in seven different populations. The populations studied were (1) Bougainville, (2) Malaita, (3) East Africa, (4) Northwest European, (5) Sioux, (6) Ifugao (Philippines), and (7) Japanese. The hair form variables included (1) average diameter, (2) nature of the medulla, (3) scale count, (4) kinking, (5) average curvature, (6) ratio of maximum to minimum curvature, (7) crimp, (8) ratio of natural to straight length. Results demonstrated that African and Melanesian populations have significantly different quantitative hair form traits, particularly with respect to the regularity of curvature.

Other Types of Information

In addition to the foregoing information, it may be possible to ascertain certain other features from a hair sample. It often is possible to determine the manner in which the hair was removed. Hair which has been cut recently will tend to have a well-defined, sharp angle on the end. As the time between cutting and removal lengthens, the ends tend to become rounder.

Hairs which have roots with a broken or ruptured sheath most likely have been torn or ripped off. If the root sheath is intact, the hair likely has merely fallen out.

Hair which has been dyed tends to show, especially under the microscope, an uneven distribution of color. Often the hair will retain its natural color near its base. Even within the dyed portion of the hair projecting above the epidermis there may be unevenly dyed patterns or patches which did not dye at all along the surface of the shaft.

Neutron Activation Analysis

In recent years, considerable interest has been generated about the use of neutron activation analysis in the positive identification of hair. Neutron activation is a technique whereby materials are irradiated and the atoms are converted into radioactive isotopes. Given the physical characteristics of the radiation, it is possible to compare the element's radioactivity with known standards.

Cornelis (1972) has summarized the requirements for the identification of hair.

1. The distribution of the analysis results as yielded by a uniform sample (governed by possible chemical treatments, counting procedures, and statistics).

2. The dispersion calculated from the analysis of several hair samples of one individual, all taken at the same time (this controls the homogeneity over one head).

3. The dispersion obtained on one individual, but with the hair being collected chronologically at successive dates (thus expressing the influence of living conditions and body intake).

4. The degree of the distribution of the trace elements in hair over a population (characterizing the individuality).

There is currently considerable controversy concerning the utilization of neutron activation analysis. The findings and views of Cornelis may be presented to summarize current status in the area:

> In conclusion the author can positively state that, with the exception of zinc, no period of time can be put forward during which the trace elements in hair remain constant (for instance within 15 per cent). . . . To sum up, it can be concluded that the trace elements present in hair are not as constant nor their concentration as specific as was suggested by the enthusiasts who introduced neutron activation analysis of hair so prematurely in court. . . . Hence the author's firm conviction that neutron activation analysis of hair, or, as a matter of fact, any other approach based on the assessment of trace elements of hair for identification purposes, is unreliable. Not only is it impossible to establish with certainty a relationship between a given hair and a suspect but it proves equally impossible to exclude beyond doubt such a relationship.

Hair as Evidence

In summary, it would be wise to consider what sorts of conclusions may be drawn from hair evidence. It should be kept in mind that a person's hair is not unique to him and that hair from one person may share identical microscopic characteristics with hair from other individuals. Therefore, it usually is not possible to state unequivocally that a sample of hair found at a scene has originated from one particular suspect. Even when the characteristics and features of the hair sample agree in all its microscopic characteristics, with all those characteristics of the hair of some suspect, hair evidence is circumstantial from an evidentiary point of view. Its subsequent importance in a case will depend on its relationship to other evidence and testimony.

On the other hand, if the hair at a scene has sufficient dissimilarities with the hair of a suspect, it would be reasonable to assume that the questioned hair did not originate from the suspect at hand.

References

Alexander, J. F.: Search for factors influencing personal identification. In Zavala, A. and Paley, J. (Eds.): *Personal Appearance Identification.* Springfield, Thomas, 1972.

Allison, H. C.: *Personal Identification.* Boston, Holbrook, 1973.

Appleyard, H. M.: *Guide to the Identification of Animal Fibres.* Leeds, Wool Industries Research Assn., 1960.

Bang, G. and Ramm, E.: Determination of age in humans from root dentin transparency. *Acta Odontol Scand, 28:3,* 1970.

Bargogna, M. and Pereira, M.: A study of absorption-elution as a method of identification of rhesus antigens in dried bloodstains. *J Forensic Sci Soc, 7:*123, 1967.

Bass, W. M.: *Human Osteology.* Columbia, Missouri Archaeological Soc., 1971.

Bates, B. P.: *I.S.Q.D.—Identification System for Questioned Documents.* Springfield, Thomas, 1970.

Baxter, P. G.: The distinction between "graphology" and "questioned document examination." *Med Sci Law, 7:*75, 1966.

Baxter, P. G.: Classification and measurement in forensic handwriting comparisons. *Med Sci Law, 13:*166, 1973.

Blackburn, D. and Caddell, W.: *The Detection of Forgery.* London, Layton, 1909.

Bloom, B. H. and Basinger, M.: On the determination of the intelligence of adults from samples of their penmanship. *J Appl Psychol, 16:*515, 1932.

Brothwell, R.: *Digging Up Bones.* London, British Museum (NH), 1972.

Camp, F. R., Kaplan, H. S., Ellis, F. R., Zmijewski, C. M., and Conte, N. F.: Tissue transplantation—the universal donor and blood group antibodies. *J Forensic Sci, 15:*500, 1970.

Camps, F. E.: *Medical and Scientific Investigations in the Christie Case.* London, Medical Publ., 1953.

Camps, F. E.: *Gradwohl's Legal Medicine.* Baltimore, Williams & Wilkins, 1968.

Candela, P. B.: Blood groups reactions in ancient human skeletons. *Am J Phys Anthropol, 21:*429, 1939.

Candela, P. B.: Blood group determination upon Minnesota and New York skeletal material. *Am J Phys Anthropol, 24:*361, 1937.

Candela, P. B.: Blood group tests on stains, mummified tissues, and cancellous bone. *Am J Phys Anthropol, 25:*187, 1939.

152

Candela, P. B.: Reliability of blood group tests on human bones. *Am J Phys Anthropol, 27*:365, 1940.

Carbonell, V. M.: Variations in the frequency of shovel-shaped incisors in different populations. In Brothwell, D. R. (Ed.): *Dental Anthropology.* London, Pergamon, 1963.

Carter, C. O.: *An ABC of Medical Genetics.* Boston, Little, 1969.

Castelnuovo-Tedesco, P.: Ratings of intelligence and personality from handwriting. *Am Psychol, 1*:455, 1946.

Charney, M.: Individual identification from human skeletal material. In Wilber, C. R. (Ed.): *Forensic Biology for the Law Enforcement Officer.* Springfield, Thomas, 1974.

Charney, M.: Disaster identification: A case in applied physical anthropology. *Tebiwa, 15*:2:66, 1972.

Charney, M.: Mistaken early man in Idaho. *Tebiwa, 15*:2:68, 1972.

Comas, J.: *Manual of Physical Anthropology.* Springfield, Thomas, 1960.

Cooke, T. D.: At 102, finger-prints prove his identity. *Identification, 44*:15, 1962.

Coombs, R. R. A. and Dodd, B.: Possible application of the principle of mixed agglutination in the identification of blood stains. *Med Sci Law, 1*:359, 1961.

Cornelis, R.: Is it possible to identify individuals by neutron activation analysis of hair? *Med Sci Law, 12*:188, 1972.

Craycroft, M. J., Camp, F. R., Jr., Ellis, F. R., Conte, N. F., McPeak, M. E., and Shirley, I. G.: The forensic testing laboratory, 1971—problems, progress and people. *USAMRL Report No. 937 (DA Project No. 3A062110A821),* 1971.

Culliford, B. J.: *The Examination and Typing of Bloodstains in the Crime Laboratory.* Washington, D.C., U.S. Dept. of Justice Law Enforcement Assistance Administration, National Institute of Law Enforcement and Criminal Justice, 1971.

Culliford, B. J. and Wraxall, B. G. D.: Haptoglobin types in dried blood stains. *Nature, 211*:872, 1966.

Cummins, H.: Attempts to alter and obliterate finger prints. *J Crim Law Criminol, 25*:982, 1935.

Cummins, H. and Midlo, C.: Palmar and plantar epidermal ridge configurations (dermatoglyphics) in European Americans. *Am J Phys Anthropol, 9*:471, 1926.

Cummins, H. and Midlo, C.: *Finger Prints, Palms and Soles.* Philadelphia, Blakiston (Reprinted 1961, New York, Dover), 1943.

Cummins, H. and Steggerda, M.: Finger prints in a Dutch family series. *Am J Phys Anthropol, 20*:19, 1935.

Dahlberg, A. A.: The dentition of the American Indian. In *The Physical Anthropology of the American Indian.* New York, The Viking Fund. 1951, p. 138.

Dankmeijer, J.: Some anthropological data on finger prints. *Am J Phys Anthropol, 23:*377.

DeVilliers, H.: *The Skull of the South African Negro.* Johannesburg, Witwatersrand U Press, 1968.

Dodd, B. E.: Some recent advances in forensic serology. *Med Sci Law, 12:*195.

Eysenck, H. J.: Graphological analysis and psychiatry: An experimental study. *Br J Psychiatry, 35:*70, 1945.

Eysenck, H. J.: Neuroticism and handwriting. *J Abnorm Psychol, 43:*94, 1948.

Faust, J. and Price, J.: A twin study of graphology. *J Biosoc Sci, 4:*379, 1972.

Federal Bureau of Investigation: *The Science of Fingerprints.* Washington, D.C., United States Government Printing Office, 1963.

Ferriman, D. G.: *Human Hair Growth in Health and Disease.* Springfield, Thomas, 1971.

Fiori, A.: Detection and identification of bloodstains. In Lindquist, F. (Ed.): *Methods of Forensic Science.* New York, Interscience Publications, 1962.

Frankenberg, M. H.: Untersuchungen uber den Nachmwis des Geschlechtschromatins an den Wurzelteilen isolierter menschlicher Harre. Diss. Bonn., 71S. *Dtsch Z Ges Gericht Med, 48:*681, 1959.

Galton, F.: *Finger Prints.* London, Macmillan, 1892.

Garn, S. M.: Types and distribution of the hair in man. *Ann NY Acad Sci, 53:*498.

Genoves, S.: Proportionality of long bones and their relation to stature among mesoamericans. *Am J Phys Anthropol, 26:*67, 1967.

Glaister, J.: *Medical Jurisprudence and Toxology,* 11th ed. Edingburgh, Livingstone, 1962.

Glocke, J. W. and Oleniewski, W. A.: Voiceprint identification in the courtroom. *J Forensic Sci, 18:*232, 1973.

Goodman, R. M. (Ed.): *Genetic Disorders of Man.* Boston, Little, 1970.

Goose, D. H.: Dental measurement: An assessment of its value in anthropological studies. In Brothwell, D. R. (Ed.): *Dental Anthropology.* London, Pergamon, 1963, p. 125.

Greenwell, M. D., Willner, A., and Kirk, P. L.: Refractive index of crown hair. *J Crim Law Criminol, 31:*746, 1941.

Grunbaum, B. W.: Recent progress in the individualization of blood and the adaptation of the Hyland crossover electrophoresis system in the identification of bloodstains. *J Forensic Sci Soc, 12:*421, 1972.

Hagan, W. E.: *Disputed Handwriting.* New York, Banks & Brothers, 1894.

Haines, D. H.: Dental identification in the Rijeka air disaster. *Forensic Sci, 1:*313, 1972.

Harris, H.: *The Principles of Human Biochemical Genetics.* Amsterdam, North Holland Publ. Co., 1970.

Harrison, W. R.: *Suspect Documents.* London, Sweet & Maxwell, 1958.

Haseeb, M. A.: Studies on human blood-stains in the Sudan. *Med Sci Law, 12:*129, 1972.

Hausman, L.: Structural characteristics of the hair of mammals. *Am Naturalist, 54:*496, 1920.

Hausman, L.: The relationships of the microscopic structural characters of human head-hair. *Am J Phys Anthropol, 8:*173, 1925.

Hausman, L.: A comparative racial study of the structural elements of human head-hair. *Am Naturalist, 59:*529, 1925.

Hausman, L.: The pigmentation of human head-hair. *Am Naturalist, 61:*545, 1927.

Heglar, R.: Paleoserology techniques applied to skeletal identification. *J Forensic Sci, 17:*358, 1972.

Helpern, M. and Wiener, A. S.: Grouping of semen in cases of rape. *Fertil Steril, 12:*551, 1961.

Holt, A. J.: *Handwriting in Psychological Interpretations.* Springfield, Thomas, 1965.

Holt, S. B.: *The Genetics of Dermal Ridges.* Springfield, Thomas, 1968.

Hooton, E. A.: *Up From the Ape.* 2nd ed. New York, Macmillan, 1946.

Howells, T. H.: A study of ability to recognize faces. *J Abnorm Psychol, 33:* 124, 1938.

Hrdlicka, A.: *Anthropometry Practical.* Philadelphia, Wistar, 1952.

Hrdy, D. and Baden, H. P.: Biochemical variation of hair keratins in man and non-human primates. *Am J Phys Anthropol, 39:*19, 1973.

Hull, C. L. and Montgomery, R. B.: An experimental investigation of certain alleged relations between character and handwriting. *Psychol Review, 26:* 63, 1919.

Hurme, V. O.: Time and sequence of tooth eruption. *J Forensic Sci, 2:*377, 1957.

Imbrie, J. A. and Wyburn, G. M.: Assessment of age, sex and height from immature human bones. *Br Med J, 1:*128, 1958.

Inbau, F. E., Moenssens, A. A., and Vitullo, L. R.: *Scientific Police Investigation.* Philadelphia, Chilton, 1972.

Johanson, G. and Saldeen, T.: The identification of burnt victims with the aid of tooth and bone fragments. *J Forensic Med, 16:*16, 1969.

Jones, A. R. and Diamond, L. K.: Identification of the Kell factor in dried blood stains. *J Forensic Med, 2:*243, 1955.

Jones, D. A.: Blood samples: probability of discrimination. *J Forensic Sci Soc, 12:*355, 1972.

Kind, S. S. and Cleevely, R. M.: The use of ammoniacal bloodstain extracts in ABO groupings. *J Forensic Sci Soc, 9:*131, 1969.

Kind, S. and Overman, M.: *Science Against Crime.* London, Aldus Books, 1972.

Kipling, Rudyard: The Ladies (a poem).

Kirk, P. L.: *Crime Investigation.* New York, Interscience, 1953.

Kirk, P. L. and Grunbaum, B. W.: Individuality of blood and its forensic significance. In Wecht, C. H. (Ed.): *Legal Medicine Annual.* New York, Appleton, 1969.

Klatsky, M.: The incidence of six anomalies of the teeth and jaws. *Hum Biol, 28:*420, 1956.

Krogman, W. M.: *The Human Skeleton in Forensic Medicine.* Springfield, Thomas, 1962.

Lane, A. B.: Effects of pose position on identification. In Zavala, A. and Paley, J. (Eds.): *Personal Appearance Identification.* Springfield, Thomas, 1972.

Lasker, G. W.: Genetic analysis of the racial traits of teeth. *Cold Spring Harbor Symp Quant Biol, 15:*191, 1950.

Leonard, D. and Zavala, A.: Electroconvulsive shock, retroactive amnesia, and the single shock method. *Science, 146:*1073, 1964.

Levitan, M. and Montagu, M. F. A.: *Textbook of Human Genetics.* New York, Oxford U Pr, 1971.

Lieberman, L. R. and Culpepper, J. T.: Words vs. objects: Comparison of free verbal recall. *Psychol Rep, 17:*983, 1965.

Lincoln, P. J. and Dodd, B. E.: Mixed agglutination as a method for the determination of A, B, and H blood groups of hair. *Med Sci Law, 8:*38, 1968.

Loftus, E.: Reconstructing memory. The incredible eyewitness. *Psychology Today, 8:*116, 1974.

Luntz, L. L. and Luntz, P.: Dental identification of disaster victims by a dental disaster squad. *J Forensic Sci, 17:*63, 1972.

MacDonell, H. L.: Interpretation of bloodstains. Physical considerations. In Wecht, C. H. (Ed.): *Legal Medicine Annual.* New York, Appleton, 1969.

Mathiak, H. A.: A key to the hairs of the mammals of Southern Michigan. *J Wildlife Management, 2:*251, 1938.

Matsunga, E., Matsuda, E., and Kumi, K. A.: Sexual variation in finger pattern size and pattern types. *Proceedings of the 8th International Congress of Anthropological and Ethnological Sciences.* Tokyo and Kyoto, 1968.

Mayer, M. V.: The hair of California mammals with keys to the dorsal guard hairs of California mammals. *Am Midl Nat, 38:*480, 1952.

McCarthy, J. F.: Some aspects of normal behavior: Their use in understanding problems encountered by document examiners. *J Forensic Sci, 20:*201, 1976.

McKern, T. W. and Stewart, T. D.: Skeletal age changes in young American males, analyzed from the standpoint of age identification. Technical Report EP-45, Quartermaster Research and Development Center, U. S. Army, Natick, 1957.

Medewar, P. B.: *The Uniqueness of the Individual.* London, Methuen, 1957.

Middleton, W. C.: The ability of untrained subjects to judge neuroticism, self-confidence, and sociability from handwriting samples. *Character Personality, 9:*227, 1941a.

Middleton, W. C.: The ability of untrained subjects to judge intelligence and age from handwriting samples. *J Appl Psychol, 25:*311, 1941b.

Milgrom, F. and Campbell, W. A.: Identification of species origin of tissues found in a sewer. *J Forensic Sci, 15:*78, 1970.

Moenssens, A. A.: *Fingerprints and the Law.* Philadelphia, Chilton, 1969.

Moenssens, A. A.: *Fingerprint Techniques.* Philadelphia, Chilton, 1971.

Moritz, A. R.: Quoted by Smith, S. and Glaister, J. in *Recent Advances in Forensic Medicine,* 2nd ed. London, Churchill, 1939, p. 110.

Morris, D.: *The Naked Ape.* New York, McGraw, 1967.

Naftali, A.: Behavior factors in handwriting identification. *J Crim Law Criminol Police Sci, 56:*528, 1965.

Newman, M. T.: Population analysis of finger and palm prints in Highland and Lowland Maya Indians. *Am J Phys Anthropol, 18:*45, 1960.

Nielsen, J. C. and Henningsen, K.: Experimental studies on the determination of the Gm groups in bloodstains. *Med Sci Law, 3:*49, 1963.

Niyogi, S. K.: A study of human hairs in forensic work. *J Forensic Med, 9:* 27, 1962.

Olivier, G.: *Practical Anthropology.* Springfield, Thomas, 1969.

Osborn, A. S.: *Questioned Documents,* 2nd ed. New York, Boyd, 1929.

Osterburg, J. W.: *The Crime Laboratory: Case Studies of Scientific Criminal Investigation.* Bloomington, Indiana U Pr, 1969.

Outeridge, R. A.: Determination of the ABO group from fingernails. *Med Sci Law, 3:*275, 1963.

Pascal, G. R. and Suttell, B.: Testing the claims of a graphologist. *J Personality, 16:*192.

Pearce, J. E.: Tales that dead men tell. *Anthropological Papers, 1:*1:1-123, No. 3537, Bureau of Research in Social Sciences Study No. 14, 1935.

Pereira, M.: The identification of MN group in dried blood stains. *Med Sci Law, 3:*268, 1963.

Pereira, M.: New techniques in forensic immunology. In Simpson, K. (Ed.): *Modern Trends in Forensic Medicine,* Vol. 2. London, Butterworths, 1967.

Pons, J.: The sexual diagnosis of isolated bones of the skeleton. *Hum Biol, 27:*12, 1955.

Pophal, R.: *Das Strichbild.* Stuttgart, verlag Thieme, 1950.

Postman, L. and Egan, J. P.: *Experimental Psychology.* New York, Harper & Brothers, 1949.

Poulson, C. J.: *The Essentials of Forensic Medicine.* Springfield, Thomas, 1965.

Prokop, O. and Uhlenbruck, G.: *Human Blood and Serum Groups,* Trans. Raven, J. L., New York, Wiley Interscience. Translation of 2nd German edition, 1966.

Rao, P. D. P.: Sexual variation in the fingerprints of Australian aborigines. *Acta Genet Med Gemellol, 211:*345, 1972.

Reynolds, E. C.: The bony pelvic girdle in early infancy, a roentgenometric study. *Am J Phys Anthropol, 3:*321, 1945.

Reynolds, E. C.: The bony pelvis in prepuberal childhood. *Am J Phys Anthropol, 5:*165, 1947.

Rosenthal, D.: *The Genain Quadruplets.* New York, Basic, 1963.

Rothwell, T. J.: The effect of storage upon the activity of phosphoglucomutase and adenylate kinase enzymes in blood samples and bloodstains. *Med Sci Law, 10:*230, 1970.

Ryder, M. L.: *Hair.* London, Arnold, 1973.

Sato, M. and Ottensooser, F.: Blood group substances in body fluids. *J Forensic Med, 14:*30, 1967.

Secord, P. F.: Studies of the relationship of handwriting to personality. *J Pers, 27:*430, 1967.

Sigh, I. P. and Bhasin, M. K.: *Anthropometry.* Delhi (India), Bharti Bhawan, 1968.

Sivaram, S.: A modified azo-dye method for identification of seminal stains. *J Forensic Sci, 15:*120, 1970.

Smith, T. L.: Determining tendencies. Second half of a classification for handwriting. *J Crim Law Criminol Police Sci, 55:*526, 1964.

Sonnemann, U. and Kernan, J. P.: Handwriting analysis: A valid tool. *Personnel, 39,* No. 6, 1962.

Spence, L. E.: Study of identifying characteristics of mammal hair. Wyo. Game and Fish Comm. Fed. Aid Wyo., Proj. No. FW-3-R-10, Job Compl. Rept., Work Plan No. 10, Job No. 2W. 121 pp., 1963.

Spence, M. A., Elston, R. C., Namboodiri, K. K. and Pollitzer, W. S.: Evidence for a possible major gene effect in absolute finger ridge count. *Hum Hered, 23:*414, 1973.

Spitz, W. U., Sopher, I. M., and DiMaio, V. J. M.: Medicolegal investigation of a bomb explosion in an automobile. *J Forensic Sci, 15:*537, 1970.

Srivastava, A. C.: The fingerprints of the Sayyads of Lucknow Uttar Pradesh. *Acta Genet Med Gemellol, 21:*337, 1972.

Stains, H. J.: Key to guard hairs of middle western fur bearers. *J Wildlife Management, 22:*95, 1958.

Stedman, R.: Human population frequencies in twelve blood groupings systems. *J Forensic Sci Soc, 12:*379, 1972.

Stern, C.: *Principles of Human Genetics.* 3rd ed. San Francisco, Freeman, 1973.

Stevens, K. N., Williams, C. E., Carbonell, J. R., and Woods, B.: Speaker authentication and identification: A comparison of spectrographic and auditory presentations of speech material. *Acoustical Soc America, 44:*1596, 1968.

Stevens, P. J.: Identification of a body by unusual means. *J Forensic Med, 13:*160, 1966.

Stewart, T. D.: Bear paw remains closely resemble human remains. *FBI Law Enforcement Bulletin, 28:*11:18, 1959.

Strong, E. K., Jr.: The effect of length of series upon recognition-memory. *Psychol Rev, 19:*447, 1912.

Sussman, L. N.: *Blood Grouping Tests.* Springfield, Thomas, 1968.

Suzuki, K. and Tsuchihashi, Y.: Personal identification by means of lip prints. *J Forensic Med, 17:*52, 1970.

Sweet, G. H. and Elvins, J. W.: Human bloodstains: Individualization by crossed electroimmunodiffusion. *Science, 192:*1012, 1976.

Thieme, F. P. and Otten, C. M.: The unreliability of blood typing aged bone. *Am J Phys Anthropol, 15:*387, 1957.

Thompson, M.W. and Bandler, E.: Finger pattern combinations in normal individuals and in Down's syndrome. *Hum Biol, 45:*563, 1973.

Thomson, A.: The sexual difference in the foetal pelvis. *J Anat Physiol, 33:* 3:359, 1899.

Thorwald, J.: *The Century of the Detective.* New York, Harcourt, Brace, and World, 1965.

Tosi, O.: Evaluation of the voiceprinting method. Report to the Michigan Department of State Police, 1967.

Tosi, O.: Speaker identification through acoustic spectography. *Comptes Rendus XIV International Congress Logopedics Phoniatrics,* Paris, 138, 1968.

Tratman, E. K.: A comparison of the teeth of people. *Dental Record* (London), *70:*31-53, 1950.

Trela, F. and Turowska, B.: ABO (H) group substances in human ear fluid. *J Forensic Sci, 6:*5, 1975.

Trotter, M. and Gleser, G. C.: Estimation of stature from long bones of American whites and Negros. *Am J Phys Anthropol, 10:*463, 1952.

Trotter, M. and Gleser, G. C.: A re-evaluation of estimation of stature taken during life and of long bones after death. *Am J Phys Anthropol, 16:*79, 1958.

Tsuchihashi, Y.: Studies on personal identification by means of lip prints. *J Forensic Sci, 3:*233, 1974.

Walker, N. F.: The use of dermal configurations in the diagnosis of mongolism. *Pediatr Clin North Am,* May, 1958, p. 531.

Wall, P. M.: *Eye-Witness Identification in Criminal Cases.* Springfield, Thomas, 1971.

Walls, H. J.: *Forensic Science.* London, Sweet and Maxwell, 1968.

Weinberg, H. M., Makin, M., Nelken, D., and Gurenitch, J.: A and B antigens in human bone tissue. *J Bone Joint Surgery, 41B:*151, 1959.

Whitehead, P. H. et al.: The examination of bloodstains by Laurell electrophoresis (antigen-antibody crossed electrophoresis). *J Forensic Sci Soc, 10:*83, 1970.

Wickelgren, W. A. and Norman, D. A.: Strength models and serial position in short-term recognition memory. *J Math Psychol, 3:*316, 1966.

Wiener, A. S., with a section by M. Shapiro: *Advances in Blood Grouping II.* New York, Grune, 1965.

Wiener, A. S.: Isoagglutinins in dried blood stains—A sensitive technique for their demonstration. *J Forensic Sci, 10:*130, 1963.

Wildman, A. B.: *The Microscopy of Animal Textile Fibres.* Leeds, Wool Industries Research Assn., 1954.

Wildman, A. B.: The identification of animal textile fibres. *J Forensic Sci Soc, 1:*1, 1961.

Williams, C. S.: Aids to the identification of mole and shrew hairs with general comments on hair structure and hair determination. *J Wildlife Management, 2:*239, 1938.

Wyatt, P. R. and Parker, W. L.: A modified method of absorption-elution of bloodstains. *Canadian Soc Forensic Sci J, 5:*119, 1972.

Yada, S., Okane, M., and Sano, Y.: Blood grouping of a single human hair by means of elution technique. *Acta Crim Jap, 32:*7, 1966a.

Yada, S., Okane, M., and Sano, Y.: Blood grouping of human hairs derived from various parts of the body. *Acta Crim Jap, 32:*173, 1966b.

Yada, S., Okane, M., and Sano, Y.: A simple method for blood grouping fingernails. *Acta Crim Jap, 32:*96, 1966c.

Yada, S., Okane, M., Sano, Y., and Fukumori, Y.: Blood grouping of eyebrows, eyelashes and vibrissae by means of the elution technique. *Acta Crim Jap, 32:*173, 1966d.

Zavala, A. and Paley, J. J.: *Personal Appearance Identification.* Springfield, Thomas, 1972.

Zavala, C., Cobo, A., and Lisker, R.: Dermatoglyphic patterns in Mexican Indian groups. *Hum Hered, 21:*394, 1971.

Zavala, R. T.: Determination of facial features used in identification. In Zavala, A. and Paley, J. (Eds.): *Personal Appearance Identification.* Springfield, Thomas, 1972.

Zmijewski, C. M. and Fletcher, J. L.: *Immunohematology,* 2nd ed. New York, Appleton, 1972.

Author Index

161

Subject Index